TAKE CONTROL OF YOUR SCOLIOSIS

ONLY YOU CAN TURN YOUR SCOLIOTIC SPINE INTO A DYNAMIC, STRONG, HEALTHY AND FLEXIBLE SPINE WITH THE HOME SPINAL ACTIVE FLEXION EXERCISES(S.A.F.E.)

THE S.A.FE. EXERCISES ARE BASED ON THE ADAM'S FORWARD BEND TEST .AND THE OBSERVATION THAT MILLIONS OF ATHLETES THAT EXERCISE DAILY HAVE STRONG HEALTHY SPINES WITHOUT ANY ABNORMAL CURVES.

BY S. ELIA

IF YOU OR YOUR CHILD HAS SCOLIOSIS…
THERE IS NO MAGIC PILL TO HELP YOU

BUT WITH THE HOME SPINAL ACTIVE FLEXION EXERCISES (S.A.F.E) DONE IN THE PRIVACY OF YOUR HOME IN YOUR OWN BED YOU WILL HAVE A GOOD CHANCE TO STOP THE PROGRESSION OF THE ABNORMAL CURVE AND EVEN REVERSE IT BACK TO NORMAL!!

NEW CLASSIFICATION OF IDIOPATHIC SCOLIOSIS BASED ON THE POSSIBLE CAUSES OF THE ABNORMAL SPINAL CURVE AND BY REMOVING THE CAUSE AND THE S.A.F.E. EXERCISES THE SPINE SHOULD BE STRONG, HEALTHY, MORE FLEXIBLE AND WITHOUT ANY ABNORMAL CURVES…..

S.ELIA

(C) 2018 BY S. ELIA ALL RIGHTS RESERVED

SCOLIOSIS IS A PREVENTABLE DISEASE
AND CAN BE PREVENTED AND TREATED
WITH
  SPINAL EXERCISES.

 MILLIONS OF ATHLETES THAT EXERCISE
    DAILY
HAVE A STRONG HEALTHY FLEXIBLE
    SPINE
WITHOUT ANY ABNORMAL CURVES

A FRESH LOOK AT WHAT CAUSES THE
IDIOPATHIC FUNCTIONAL SCOLIOSIS AND
HOME EXERCISES TO   STOP THE
PROGRESSION OF THE CURVE AND EVEN

REVERSE IT BACK TO NORMAL

THERE IS HOPE TO EVERY MOTHERS ANGUISH FOR HER CHILDS CROOKED SPINE. THERE IS HOPE TO EVERYONE THAT IS DIAGNOSED WITH SCOLIOSIS IN THE EARLY STAGES OF THIS DISEASE BUT THEY HAVE TO DO THE SPINAL EXERCISES!

FOR ALL THOSE WHO ARE DIAGNOSED WITH SCOLIOSIS, DAILY EXERCISES AT HOME WILL TAME THEIR ABNORMAL SPINAL CURVES ,STOP THE PROGRESSION OF SCOLIOSIS AND GET A HEALTHY, FLEXIBLE STRONG SPINE.

Scoliosis is the million dollar question? How to prevent it and how to stop the progression of the abnormal spinal curve with home exercises! And the answer is THE SPINAL ACTIVE FLEXION. EXERCISES!!(S.A.F.E.)

IF YOU ARE A HEALTH PROFESSIONAL TREATING PEOPLE WITH SCOLIOSIS YOU WILL GET BETTER RESULTS FOR THEIR CONDITION IF YOU ENCOURAGE THEM TO DO THE SPINAL EXERCISES AT HOME……….

Disclaimer:

This book is for information ONLY and is not intended to serve as medical advice. Anyone seeking specific advice or assistance should consult his or her doctor. If they do not like the advice of their doctor they should seek a second opinion from another doctor. You should always work with the advise and blessing of your trusted doctor.

THE AUTHOR

S.ELIA

DEDICATION:

I Dedicate this book to all those people that will do my designed spinal active flexion exercises(S.A.F.E.) daily and get a strong, healthy, flexible spine and stop the progression of their abnormal spinal curve, the so called IDIOPATHIC SCOLIOSIS and even reverse it back to normal, and above all have a healthier life.

It is also dedicated to all those mothers that worry about their kid's health when they are first diagnosed with scoliosis and by encouraging and supervise their youngsters to do THE S.A.F.E. exercises daily, will give them hope and eliminate their anguish and frustration when they see their kids getting better and have a healthy, strong and flexible spine

It is also dedicated to all those health professionals that diagnose and treat people with scoliosis giving them hope and relief for their suffering.

S.ELIA

TABLE OF CONTENTS

1) PROLOGUE

2) WHAT IS SCOLIOSIS

3) HISTORY OF SCOLIOSIS

4) POSSIBLE CAUSES OF SCOLIOSIS AND SUGGESTED NEW NAMES FOR THE NOW KNOWN IDIOPATHIC SCOLIOSIS.

5) SIGNS AND SYMPTOMS OF SCOLIOSIS

6) DIAGNOSIS OF SCOLIOSIS AND POSSIBLE NEW NAMES FOR THE NOW KNOWN, "IDIOPATHIC SCOLIOSIS"

7) SUGGESTED TREATMENTS OF SCOLIOSIS

8) REASONING FOR THE DEVELOPMENT AND DESIGN OF THE HOME EXERCISES (S.A.F.E.) SPINAL ACTIVE FLEXION EXERCISES

9) DESCRIPTION OF THE S.A.F.E. EXERCISES

10) SUMMARY OF THE DAILY ROUTINE OF THE (S.A.F.E) SPINAL ACTIVE FLEXION EXERCISES

11) EXPECTED RESULTS

12) RESEARCH IS NEEDED

13) PREVENTION

14) THINGS TO DO THAT ARE GOOD FOR YOUR SPINE

15) THINGS TO AVOID THAT ARE BAD FOR YOUR SPINE

16) KEEP A DAILY DIARY TO DOCUMENT YOUR PROGRESS AND MOTIVATE YOU TO KEEP EXERCISING

17) IF YOU OR YOUR CHILD HAS SCOLIOSIS

18) IF YOU ARE A HEALTH PROFESSIONAL TREATING PEOPLE WITH SCOLIOSIS

19) CONCLUSION

20) EPILOGUE

21) REFERENCES

CHAPTER ONE

PROLOGUE

I write this book mainly for all the mothers and their youngsters that are first diagnosed with scoliosis and were told" to wait and see how the abnormal spinal curve, the scoliosis, will develop in six months, a year Etc…" The wait and see approach is not good enough and most of the time we know what will happen, the scoliosis gets worse. Instead they should stop whatever is causing their abnormal curve and start corrective exercises to stop the progression of the scoliosis and even reverse it back to its normal straight position.

There are many books about scoliosis which describe what scoliosis is and what the available treatments are. However all authors describe the scoliosis as idiopathic, that there is no known cause of the abnormal spinal curve and that there is nothing to do about it when is diagnosed until it is time to use braces and finally have surgery to stabilize the spine with rods and spinal fusion. I am sure the doctors do the best they can with what they know and they do a good job in stabilizing the spine with rods and fusion however the patients lost the normal function of the spine.

For years, I and a lot of other people, were convinced that scoliosis was due to poor posture, slouching, and bad sitting habits, and still think they cause scoliosis and other health risks.

The so called Idiopathic scoliosis occur during the growing years of the kids, it affects about 2-3% of the youngsters and affects more the girls than the boys and that made me thinking why is that? For years I was wondering why more girls had scoliosis than the boys, until One day while watching kids play in the neighborhood park, I had the AHA MOMENT.

Young kids mostly girls were lifting other younger kids and holding them on one side of their bodies and carrying them around. So I figured out that if kids do this on a daily basis with their younger siblings, cousins, nephews etc that's HOW most of the kids get their scoliosis. So I renamed the idiopathic scoliosis in youngsters "THE KIDS LIFTING BABIES SCOLIOSIS " OR BABYSITTING JUVENILE SCOLIOSIS" When they baby-sit, PLAY or take care of babies.

The answer might be simple and the idiopathic scoliosis is not idiopathic anymore but it is a serious cause that nobody paid any attention to it before. Who could think that the idiopathic scoliosis is caused with kids lifting other kids while playing and having fun? We give girls dolls to play with and when they are older they like to play with LIVE HEAVY babies, sibling, nieces, nephews or the neighbors' babies. sometimes babies might be very heavy and if they have access to these kids daily for a long period of time AND THEY LIFT THEM AND CARRYING THEM AROUND ON ONE SIDE OF THEIR BODIES that's where their scoliosis start……………. BINGO!!!!!

Another reason why girls have scoliosis more often than the boys is that the girls like to hug more than the boys and if they hug the wrong way this will be the beginning of their scoliosis. Even when they start dating and they walk with their dates they lean on one side towards their dates and if they do that day in and day out this might cause some problem to their spine. But the main reason that the girls have scoliosis more often than the boys, is the lifting heavy kids and carrying them around………..

That is why girls have scoliosis more than the boys do.

The motherhood instinct.

CHAPTER TWO

WHAT IS SCOLIOSIS

SCOLIOSIS IS A SPINAL DISORDER THAT CAUSES AN ABNORMAL CURVE OF THE SPINE TO THE SIDE ,AFFECTS ABOUT 2-3% OF THE POPULATION CAN OCCUR AT ANY AGE BUT MOSTLY BETWEEN THE AGES OF 8 AND 20 and affects MORE girls than boys. The spine or as otherwise known THE VERTEBRAL COLUMN has a total of 33 vertebrae ,7 in the cervical region ,that's the neck bones, 12 vertebrae in the thoracic region, 5 in the lumbar region , that's the low back, 5 sacral vertebrae which are fused together and they form the base of the spine, and 4 coccygeal vertebrae which are also fused together . The spine with the 24 vertebrae from the sacrum to the base of the skull forms a hollow canal which encloses and protects THE SPINAL CORD which is an extension of the brain… From the spinal cord arise the spinal nerves and the nerves leave the spinal canal through a small opening called the inter vertebral foramen, a total of 31 pairs of spinal nerves which supply nerve energy to all parts of the body. .The abnormal curve called Scoliosis changes the size of the inter vertebral foramen , the opening from which the spinal nerves arise from the spinal cord, and puts pressure on the spinal cord and nerves causing pain and interruption to the nerve supply of the affected nerves.. Scoliosis affects the skeletal system the spine, ribs, and pelvis and it also affects the brain ,central nervous system that is housed in the spinal canal , and the body's hormonal system and can damage major organs including the heart and lungs In other words the abnormal curve called SCOLIOSIS affects the functions of the whole body .

SCOLIOSIS IS CLASSIFIED EITHER AS STRUCTURAL IN WHICH THE CURVE IS FIXED OR FUNCTIONAL IN WHICH THE BONES OF THE SPINE ARE NORMAL. BOTH STRUCTURAL AND FUNCTIONAL SCOLIOSIS IS TRYING TO STRAIGHTEN WHEN BENDING FORWARD. (ADAM 'S TEST)

The abnormal curve of the spine is usually S or C in shape and it can be mild or severe. Mild scoliosis does not cause problems but if untreated leads to severe scoliosis causing aesthetic and serious health problems .

The normal human spine is straight when you see it from the back or the front but the spine with scoliosis has abnormal curvatures to the side .

When you x-ray the scoliosis spine you will see a sideways curve which can be measure with the COBB angle method and can vary from a mild a few degrees up to many degrees.
The bigger the COBB ANGLE the worse the scoliosis is.

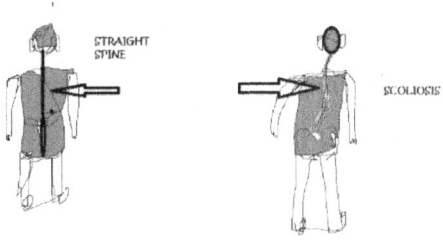

Scoliosis spines are seen only in humans and very rarely in animals.

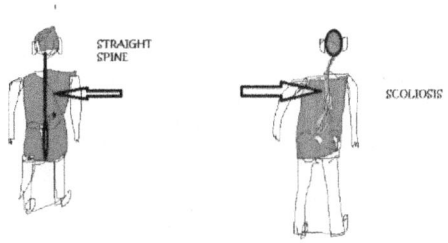

CHAPTER THREE

HISTORY OF SCOLIOSIS

The ancient Greeks had a saying «νους υγιης εν σωματι υγιη«
"A HEALTHY MIND IN A HEALTHY BODY".
They recognized the importance of a healthy strong body and they were spending hours to exercise to

have a good strong body. They organize the Olympics and other regional games every year to show off their achievement in the development of physical abilities. They were training their youths to be both physical and mentally strong.

Despite all their efforts there were some cases of scoliosis due to injuries or some pathology and Hippocrates the father of medicine was the first to recognize and describe the condition. He devised some contraptions to treat the scoliosis with some of his ideas are still used to-day by some trying to straighten the abnormal curve.

The Spartans in ancient Greece had the best trained soldiers of that era, and hey started the training of their soldiers at age 7. Their daily routine was to swim in the river Eurotas, strenuous exercises in the art of fighting and other exercises. The body of these youngsters was strong and flexible and they had no scoliosis or other spinal problems.
This might be an indication that with daily exercises, swimming and other exercises, keeps the spine healthy, strong, and can prevent scoliosis.

From the ancient time of Hippocrates the father of medicine till now, people tried to correct the abnormal curvature of the spine called SCOLIOSIS. UNFORTUNATELY they have not invented any magic pill YET to correct the abnormal curvature of the spine.

They managed to find the cause of scoliosis from infections such as polio and tuberculosis and other pathological conditions, and by treating properly those diseases they manage to eliminate the scoliosis that were caused by those diseases. They had success in eliminating poliomyelitis and treat tuberculosis that were causing pathological scoliosis but other forms of scoliosis are still a mystery and researchers are searching to find the cause of scoliosis.

So far they did not come up with a cause and they simply call it idiopathic scoliosis, which means they do not know the cause.

Every year governments and other organizations spend millions of dollars in research to find the cause and treatment of scoliosis. The real question is, have they been looking at the right place? I.e. The youngsters that are affected with scoliosis and their lifestyle habits and environment?

They tried hard devising braces and expensive treatments but still the quest remains. Surgery with the insertion of still rods has some success to correct it but the patients lost the normal function of the spine and there are many risks associated with any surgery.

Despite the advancement of modern medicine, in the scientific community the cause of scoliosis remain a mystery and they have not found a way to prevent or a cure that is reliable, risk free for the patients.

They fail to correct the scoliosis because they did not know the cause or how the scoliosis starts and if you do not know the cause of a disease you can not treat it successfully. That's why they called it idiopathic, of unknown cause. First you have to find the cause of the disease eliminates the cause and the patient will get well, and of course you have to have the full co-operation of the patient.

CHAPTER FOUR

POSSIBLE CAUSES OF SCOLIOSIS AND SUGGESTED NEW NAMES FOR THE NOW

KNOWN IDIOPATHIC SCOLIOSIS

The cause of scoliosis. Let's examine the possible cause of the abnormal sideways curve of the spine called scoliosis or simply "crooked spine."

Scoliosis has many causes:

1) It can be due to severe trauma and this is a medical emergency and it is treated in hospitals by the specialist and it is not going to be discussed here

.2) Due to some pathology, tumors, collapse discs, osteoporosis etc. it is best treated by the medical specialists and is not going to be discussed here.

3) The IDIOPATHIC SCOLIOSIS Which STARTS SLOWLY and progresses with time. It is called idiopathic because they do not know what is causing it. This is the most common scoliosis affecting the spine of million of youngsters age 7 to 18 , the growing years and some of them will end up having major surgeries to correct their spines and loose their spinal flexibility.

There are many types of scoliosis depending on the age of the individual but we are going to talk about the idiopathic scoliosis that occurs to babies the so called INFANTILE IDIOPATHIC SCOLIOSIS which affect babies 0-3 years of age, AND ADOLESCENT IDIOPATHIC SCOLIOSIS which affects youngsters age 8 to 18. Here were are going to examine the possible causes of this so called idiopathic scoliosis, examine ways to prevent it and with home exercises to stop the progression of the abnormal curve and even correct it when it is in the early stages, provided the patients will follow the instructions to stop doing what is causing their scoliosis and do the exercises religiously daily for ever or at least when they are adults.

THE CAUSE OF INFANTILE idiopathic scoliosis which occurs from 0-3 years of age. Most of the authors on the infantile scoliosis they classified it as idiopathic with unknown cause.

However I have a different opinion and I strongly believe that infantile scoliosis has a definite cause and that's the way they position the baby while sleeping, sitting or they hold the baby. If the baby was born normal and after a while a scoliosis appears on the baby, if the baby had no falls or other unforeseen accident, then the cause of the scoliosis is due to the way they have the baby to sleep. If the baby sleeps on the stomach, or always on one side, will have scoliosis in the neck region and low back AND EVEN some face and skull malformation. The baby's skull is very soft after birth and it can easily malformed if the baby sleeps in one position for long periods of time. If the mother or the care givers carry the baby on one side of their body ALL THE TIME, the baby will have a C type scoliosis. The mother might also develop some scoliosis or pains and aches in her spine. Because I think the cause of the infantile scoliosis is due to the positioning of the baby by the care givers

I give this type of idiopathic scoliosis a new name

POSITIONAL INFANTILE SCOLIOSIS

to be distinguished from other forms of infantile scoliosis such as traumatic, or due to some other recognizable cause, infections, or pathology etc.

When we give this type of scoliosis a name POSITIONAL INFANTILE SCOLIOSIS, with a known cause, the BAD POSITIONS they put the baby, instead of idiopathic scoliosis of unknown cause, every one will know how to treat the condition the right way: Remove the cause that causes the scoliosis, the BAD POSITIONING.

If the POSITIONAL INFANTILE SCOLIOSIS is recognized early by the parents and the pediatrician that looks after the baby and give the mother the right instructions the infantile positional scoliosis will reverse to a normal spine. If the pediatrician gives the mother "the regular wait and see what happens approach "and they continue the same old routine with bad positions, the baby will have spinal and health problems later on. The scoliosis will get worse with time might even need corrective surgery.

The correct instructions should be, to reverse the old position they were positioning the baby. If the baby was sleeping on his stomach, now should be sleeping on his back, and if the baby was sleeping always on the right side now should be sleeping on his left side until the spine, skull and the face return to normal. Later on when the baby starts to crawl they should encourage the baby to crawl as much as possible, as crawling tends to correct the spine and that's why animals that walk on their four feet they do not get scoliosis.
If you get the baby some swimming lessons that will help a lot.

Adolescent IDIOPATHIC SCOLIOSIS which is the most common scoliosis affecting youngsters 8 to 18 years of age is called idiopathic because they did not figured out what the cause is YET............... I happened to believe that adolescent idiopathic scoliosis has a few recognizable causes which has to do with the lifestyle of the youngsters and possible micro trauma which was not diagnosed properly.

If the positional infantile scoliosis (the so called infantile idiopathic scoliosis) is not recognized early and treated properly the abnormal spinal curve (scoliosis) will continue to get worse over the years and by the time the kids reach their teens might need surgical intervention to stabilize the spine. When the scoliosis starts after the age of 7 the cause is due to bad posture, slouching while playing video games and television watching and sitting in a crooked way to read and write at home and school carrying heavy backs on one side of their body over a period of long time and straining and micro trauma in the pelvis sacrum spinal joints.

Most types of the scoliosis starts in the low back area at the lumbar sacral bones.
I remember one of my classmates who was sitting on the desk in front of me and he had the bad habit to lean forward put his left elbow on the desk and bend his body to the left close to the book he was reading or writing and he eventually got a crooked spine (mild scoliosis) to the left.

I am sure that many kids that have such bad habits will develop scoliosis eventually. if the doctor that first diagnoses this type of scoliosis advises the child and the parents " TO WAIT AND SEE WHAT HAPPENS APPROACH " and the child continues his bad sitting habits, his spine will get worse and eventually might need surgery to correct the scoliosis. I rename this type of idiopathic scoliosis to BAD HABITS POSTURAL SCOLIOSIS, OR JUST POSTURAL SCOLIOSIS, because its cause is the bad posture habits and when they do it day in day out they will develop a crooked spine. In the early stages this type of scoliosis is reversible provided that the kids stop the bad posture slouching habits and do the right exercises which I will describe under exercises for the treatments of scoliosis.

And finally the MYSTERY of scoliosis that affect more girls than boys it is caused when the young girls baby sit or play for long periods of time with babies, siblings, cousins nephews neighbors kids , lifting them and holding them in their arms either on left or right side .It is usually starting slowly but if they continue to do this for a long period of time the scoliosis will get worse,.

I name this type of scoliosis BABYSITTING JUVENILE SCOLIOSIS (playing, lifting, babysitting and taking care Of younger kids).

The doctor should ask specific questions when the scoliosis diagnosis is made to find the real cause of this not so unusual type of scoliosis. Simply ask them if they have access to babies, siblings, nephews, cousins or other kids and if they baby-sit, play and spend long hours holding the babies.

The rest of the idiopathic scoliosis in that age group is probably caused by micro trauma, sprain or strain in their spine or the pelvis, sacrum ,spine , which was not diagnosed to be treated properly, as the youngsters might have not complained.

Just think about for a moment : how many times kids and adults slip and fall on their buttock while walking or playing , they get some pain in their low back , but they fail to see a doctor for diagnosis and treatment if necessary. This might be the beginning of some type of scoliosis, mild or severe if not recognized and treated properly.

When there is a strain or sprain in the lower back and pelvic joints it might create a false short leg on one side and this in return if not treated properly will cause mild spinal curve in the lower back and eventually while the body tries to straighten out creates a new curve in the thoracic region and that's the making of abnormal S CURVE Type of scoliosis.

This type of scoliosis I will name it as

TRAUMATIC COMPENSATORY SCOLIOSIS

due to a false short leg, and my guess is that's the cause of the majority of the so called idiopathic scoliosis.

If you examine these patients while lying face down you will notice that they have an apparent short leg and if you ask them they probably tell you that they did have a fall, strain or low back pain which they did not seek treatment……..if not they might have a true short leg that is causing their scoliosis and you have to fix that with a shoe lift on that side in order to have any success in treating their scoliosis. If a true short leg is causing S type of scoliosis I name this as:

SHORT LEG COMPENSATORY SCOLIOSIS.

Now that we know what causes each type of scoliosis, instead of calling it IDIOPATHIC, we will try to eliminate the cause and with the full cooperation of the patients their scoliosis should improve or even reverse. Without the patients cooperation no treatment can be successfully.

We took the so called IDIOPATHIC SCOLIOSIS, with no known cause, we examined the possible causes and re-classify it according to its cause with a known OR possible cause. And I have reclassified to:

1)POSITIONAL INFANTILE SCOLIOSIS (from the old infantile idiopathic scoliosis which is caused when the mother or care giver hold the babies on one side or place the babies in one side when they sleep.)

2)BAD HABITS POSTURAL ADOLESCENT

SCOLIOSIS OR JUST POSTURAL ADOLESCENT SCOLIOSIS (from the old idiopathic adolescent scoliosis ,which is caused by bad postural habits in their daily lives.)

3)BABYSITTING SCOLIOSIS (from the old juvenile idiopathic scoliosis that affect more girls than boys and the cause is babysitting or lifting and playing with babies)

4)TRAUMATIC COMPENSATORY SCOLIOSIS (from the old idiopathic juvenile scoliosis)this type of scoliosis is due to untreated strains, sprains, or other injuries to the low back and pelvic joints. or by just kids being kids fooling around or playing practical jokes or even bending down to pick their ball and can get a low back strain .)

5)SHORT LEG COMPENSATORY SCOLIOSIS (From the old idiopathic juvenile scoliosis, when there is a true short leg .)

In conclusion There is always a Cause of scoliosis.

There is no such thing as idiopathic scoliosis, there is always a cause from the time of birth to adulthood .

If the babies are born naturally with no human intervention or instrumentation they have a normal spine. The danger of developing a scoliosis spine starts right after birth with the way the parents or other caregivers will care for the child.

ONCE THE SCOLIOTIC CURVATURE STARTS TO DEVELOP IT WILL CONTINUE TO GET WORSE UNLESS THERE IS an intervention to find out what's causing the abnormal curvature.

They should examine all possible cause from an injury from lifting or carrying something heavy to slouching. The patient should be instructed how to sit properly, sit straight, stand tall, avoid lifting heavy objects and bad posture, avoid sitting in a crooked position watching TV for long time.

CHAPTER FIVE

SIGNS AND SYMPTOMS OF SCOLIOSIS

People with scoliosis might have pain in the low back, neck and shoulder blades and sometimes in the early stages, the scoliosis can be without pain.

When the scoliosis is severe with the spine severely crooked it can cause serious health problems affecting the lungs, heart and other the parts of the body .

People with scoliosis have uneven shoulders, one shoulder blade is more prominent than the other, and have a rib hump One hip higher than the other uneven hips arms or leg lengths.

Sometimes other people, family friends and classmates notice the scoliosis first

CHAPTER SIX

DIAGNOSIS OF SCOLIOSIS

AND SUGGESTED NEW NAMES FOR THE NOW KNOWN " IDIOPATHIC SCOLIOSIS"

Anybody can see a crooked spine when the abnormal curve is severe , but a definite diagnosis is made by taking a full x ray of the spine with the patient standing, AP and lateral views and measuring the COBB angle to see how bad the abnormal curve is.
The greater the COBB angle the worse the scoliosis is.

There is also a simple test the" ADAMS TEST" by asking the patient to bend forward with the knees straight to see if there is an abnormality on one side of the spine(the curve of the scoliosis) a rib hump where the ribs on one side protrude.

To diagnose
the positional infantile scoliosis ,
is done by physical examination of the baby's spine

and face and if there are indications of an abnormal spinal curve to take x rays to confirm the diagnosis. You will also have to do detective work and ask specific questions of the mother or others who care for the baby to differentiate if it is positional or has other cause such as trauma during delivery with instrumentation ,a fall at home or even some underlying pathology or negligence. These are the questions to ask the mother or caregivers..

1) was the delivery normal without instrumentations? In a difficult delivery with the use of instruments there is a possibility for the baby to sustain injuries to his neck , head and spine and cause the scoliosis(traumatic infantile scoliosis), wry neck, even cerebral palsy..

2) what's the position the baby usually sleep? a)face up on his back   b) right side all the time   c)left side all the time   d) not the same position   e) face down with the neck twisted to one side. different positions can cause different changes

3) is the baby sleeping well or does he wake up and cry often? (Waking up and crying might be an indication that the position the baby sleeps causes some strain and pain)

4) any changes to his face and skull appearance since birth? When was the first time noticed the skull and face changes? any pictures of the baby at

different intervals to notice any face abnormalities. pictures will show if there is a change from the time of birth. Change to the babies face is indicative that the baby sleep one side all the time or face down.

5) any accidental fall of the baby? if yes was the baby examined by a doctor? what did he say? Falls can cause injuries to the baby's spine

6) are there any siblings or other kids that hold and play with the baby? if yes how often? kids might have accidentally dropped or injured the baby.

7) did the baby had a serious infection or serious illness that required hospitalization for a long time? If the child had an illness might have effected his spine.

8) who cares for the baby? The mother or somebody else? Very important to know, if someone else is caring for the baby, might be abuse and negligence.

From the answers you get, you will have an idea if it is POSITIONAL INFANTILE SCOLIOSIS, where the baby sleeps on same side all time or has other cause such as a fall, negligence or from other cause.

To diagnose the

BAD HABITS POSTURAL SCOLIOSIS
you have to take x-rays AP and lateral to identify the abnormal curve and do detective work about their lifestyle and postural habits .
You have to have a detailed case history and the lifestyle of the youngster, how they sleep, how the sit at school, at home and when they watch television or play video games, if they exercise , how often and what sports they play.
If they have bad sitting habits , sleep face down, play no sports and do not exercise and had no history of injury, then it is BAD HABITS POSTURAL SCOLIOSIS or simply POSTURAL SCOLIOSIS. Usually the bad habits postural scoliosis is C TYPE SCOLIOSIS.

THE BABYSITTING FUNCTIONAL SCOLIOSIS

is diagnosed from the case history and x-rays. The x-rays confirm the crooked spine and the case history will differentiate it from any other scoliosis.
.The youngsters with this type of scoliosis will have access to babies either babysitting or playing with them for long periods of time lifting them holding them etc.
This type of scoliosis it can be either C type or S Type scoliosis .They might have strain or sprain in the low back , sacroiliac joints from lifting the babies CAUSING AN ABNORMAL CURVE in the low back and a compensatory curve in the thoracic region from holding the babies .or just C

curve from holding the babies on one side of their bodies. Even boys can get this type of scoliosis when they have access to babies and they lift, or hold babies.

The definite diagnosis of any abnormal curvature is made by x-rays and then you have to do detective work to differentiate and find the real cause.

The above causes that cause scoliosis mentioned are the most common causes of the so called idiopathic juvenile scoliosis , but I am sure there are a lot more causes of scoliosis, such as unreported and untreated injuries from horsing around, playing practical jokes or injuries from playing certain contact sports such as football, soccer , wrestling and even injuries from playing on a trampoline etc. it might be very difficult to find the cause that causes scoliosis in such cases especially
if the youngsters do not remember such injuries. In such cases the term **IDIOPATHIC SCOLIOSIS** might be justified, until the real or possible cause is recognized .
 there is always a cause but the youngsters do no remember and did not report it .

4) to diagnose the

TRAUMATIC COMPENSATORY JUVENILE SCOLIOSIS

you have to do detective work to see if the patient remembers and had an untreated injury.

To confirm the diagnosis you take x-rays to see that the curve starts at the lumbar sacral area and one ileum is higher than the other causing a functional false short leg. And when you press on the pelvic joints and low lumbar joints you might elicit pain.
You also have to measure the leg length to make sure that is not a true short leg.

5)The SHORT LEG COMPENSATORY SCOLIOSIS
is diagnosed by taking x rays to verify the abnormal curve of scoliosis and the pelvis to be lower on one side and the hip lower than the other one. When you measure the leg lengths' you will find that one leg is shorter than the other. A true short leg.

CHAPTER SEVEN

SUGGESTED TREATMENTS OF SCOLIOSIS

There are many treatments for scoliosis. Some of them are good some of them so-so and some risky and dangerous, like the corrective surgery and the use of rods, although I must say that in many cases it is absolutely necessary and sometimes with good results. Most children when they are first diagnosed with a mild scoliosis they are told to wait and see how the curve will develop in six months to a year without any treatments or advice.

To "the wait and see approach

I have to agree with Dr.. 'John H. Moe 1905-

1988 a University of Minnesota orthopedic surgeon, who founded the Scoliosis Research Society in 1966 and he began a "do not delay" campaign for scoliosis, and he wrote " procrastination was the most pernicious problem in idiopathic scoliosis and sad to see a child come with a severe curve requiring surgery with X-rays taken many years before showing a mild curve that could have been easily treated with a brace.46'Dangerous Curve" campaign

When the abnormal curve gets worse in six months or a year they advice them to use a brace for a period of time and if that does not help the scoliosis they have surgery to fuse the spine and use rods to straighten the spine.

I am not familiar with braces used to treat scoliosis and I do not know what rate of success they have so I have no opinion whether to use a brace or not.

I Saw Some pictures of those braces and they look bulky and uncomfortable .

The idea of bracing probably came from the same idea that the farmers use straight sticks to support their young seedling trees so that their

trunk grows straight. It protects the young trees from the elements of nature and works perfectly for the young trees but the trees do not have to go anywhere and just stand there until they grow and their trunk is strong and straight.
 It is a great idea for the trees but not so for the youngsters, they have to move and do things which is very uncomfortable and unable to do the usual things which we take for granted that we should be able to do, like bending over to tie your shoes, or go to the washroom etc. plus there is pressure on certain area of their bodies ,trying to keep the spine straight and every time they move their bodies is uncomfortable and can even cause some irritation on the skin where the pressure is applied.

Anyway if some youngsters can put up with all that and do not cheat, they might see some benefits and their scoliosis will stop the progression and might even avoid the rods and spinal fusion.

 Instead of bulky and heavy braces in mild scoliosis I might recommend a soft lumbar sacral support to protect the low back from further injuries , and spinal exercises to get stronger muscles and more flexible spine .
 <u>With the spinal active exercises which I designed they will also get re-alignment of their pelvic and hip joints to restore normal</u>

function to those joints.

Treatments with corrective exercises should start as soon as possible after the diagnosis of scoliosis is made to stop the progression of the abnormal curve.
Some of the conservative treatments such as physiotherapy, the schroth method and others that have limited success may be due to the fact that they fail to teach the patient what to avoid while getting treatments or what they should do at home.

Because if you do the exercises for 30 minutes or an hour, trying to push the spine to its normal position and the patient goes home and keeps doing what they have been doing to cause the scoliosis in the first place, it's obvious that they will put their spine to a scoliosis state AGAIN and the treatment has no effect

For anybody who attempts to correct the scoliotic spine they must first have the full co-operation of the patient and the patient follows all the recommendations of the treating practitioner. If they do not have their full co-operation.

NO TREATMENT OR EXERCISE

will correct the abnormal curvature if they fail to give instructions to the patient what to do after the treatment and what to avoid in between treatments ,again the treatment will not be effective or have lasting effects.

Many of these conservative treatments are expensive and many times inconvenient as the patients have to travel long distances or they have to stay in an inpatient intensive rehabilitation program. If the patients have some correction during their stay or while getting treatments and when they go home start doing whatever they were doing to get the scoliosis in the first place, they will end up with the same old curvature or even worse.

Since I have no idea what type of success the physiotherapy and other therapies get and I have no idea what instruction they give to their patients during and after treatments, I cannot say anything about those therapies. If the patients are satisfied with their treatment and see improvements in their condition its up to the patients to say if this or that therapy is good or not and stick with it or not.

Besides all the known therapies including surgery , are treating the scoliosis as **IDIOPATHIC WITH UNKNOWN CAUSE** , so in reality they treat the symptoms of scoliosis and not the cause because they do not know the cause. If you do not know the cause of a disease you cannot treat it properly and remove the cause.

That's the reason why I reclassified the idiopathic scoliosis into five new names according to what is causing each type of scoliosis ..
In every type of scoliosis you have to remove the cause first and with the proper exercises the spinal muscles will get stronger and have an effect on the spinal curves including scoliosis.

Suggested Treatments of the

INFANTILE POSITIONAL SCOLIOSIS :

Treatments, or rather exercises should start as soon as possible, with the blessing of the attending doctor, when a diagnosis is made ".The wait and see approach" is not good enough and dangerous for the patient.
The mother or the care giver of the baby should switch the usual positions that the baby was lying sleeping or holding the baby. If the baby was sleeping all the time on his left side now should

be placed on his right side or on his back. if they were holding the baby on the right side now switch to left. When they bathe or change the baby they should place the baby on his back and encourage the baby to move his arms and legs.

Exercises are good for everyone including babies.

When the baby is able to crawl encourage him to crawl as much as possible. Encourage the babies to sleep on their back and never face down. when they are older give them swimming lessons and exercises on a monkey bar.

It is very important to recognize and treat the positional infantile scoliosis early. If left unrecognized, undiagnosed and untreated ,it will get worse with time and might need corrective surgeries in the future.

And I quote from the dangerous curve Dr. john H .Moe 1905-1988 who began a "do not delay" campaign for scoliosis, and wrote "it is sad to see a child come with a severe curve requiring surgery with X-rays taken many years before showing a mild curve that could have been easily treated with a brace."

Besides the INFANTILE POSITIONAL SCOLIOSIS is the easiest to recognize and treat successfully since it is in the early stage and kids respond better to treatments as they do not have to do much, the adults that care for the baby do all that is needed.

N.B. I watch some videos on infantile scoliosis where they were applying braces or casts on the kids and I must say that I was disappointed. I am just wondering if those casts and braces are causing more harm than good. Kids at that age should be encouraged to move and exercise and not be confined in a cast or brace that cause stiffness and weakness to the muscles from inactivity.

According to the doctor who made the video the success rate of the casting and bracing are about 25 percent and some of the kids that had casting and braces they end up in surgery later on. That is not very good results and a lot of trouble that kids go through.

Instead of casts and heavy braces they should give their mother a prescription for exercises and encourage their mother to let their kids move around more with crawling, running, swimming , the monkey bar exercises and of course the S.A.F.E. exercises. By the time they are ready to go school their abnormal curve should disappear with the exercises.

Suggested Treatments for the bad habits POSTURAL SCOLIOSIS OR JUST

JUVENILE POSTURAL SCOLIOSIS

should start immediately as soon as the diagnosis is made. Remove the cause, which are bad habits. and emphasize that the bad habits they have BAD affects on their spine and unless they change their habits the scoliosis will get worse and they may end up having corrective surgery with spinal fusion and rods in their spine.

Give them instructions how to sit when reading, writing, watch television and how to lift properly and of course to start the S.A.F.E. (spinal active flexion exercises), along with the monkey bar exercises and swimming whenever they have the time.

The suggested treatments for
BABYSITTING JUVENILE FUNCTIONAL SCOLIOSIS

is by removing the cause which is the association with babies, with advising the patient to stop babysitting, lifting or carrying around any babies and the same instructions as with postural scoliosis , and the S.A.F.E. EXERCISES , monkey bar exercises, holding the monkey bar with both hands and swinging back and forth, creating natural traction of the spine with the weight of their body, swimming and other sport activities. They should start exercising as soon as the diagnosis is made.

" The wait and see approach is not a good option. "If they Keep babysitting and lifting heavy babies the scoliosis will get worse AND MIGHT NEED CORRECTIVE SURGERY!

The suggested treatment for

TRAUMATIC COMPENSATORY JUVENILE SCOLIOSIS

is more difficult to treat but by taking care of the low back by using an elastic support for the lumbar sacral area, proper lifting instructions, good postural habits and the S.A.F.E. EXERCISES they should see some improvement.

The elastic support is removed when exercising.

The monkey bar exercises and swimming should also help.

They should avoid any rough contact sport, like wrestling, hockey and football.

The suggested treatment for the

TRUE SHORT LEG JUVENILE SCOLIOSIS

is treated by removing the cause which is the short leg.

This is the type of scoliosis that people affected with polio had when one of their legs was affected. They should have a heel or shoe lift in the shoe of the affected SHORT leg.

With the S.AF.E. EXERCISES , the monkey bar and swimming exercises should see some improvement in their spinal curve.

Basically to have an improvement in the curve of scoliosis, any type of scoliosis, you have to remove the cause that is causing the scoliosis, whatever the cause is, and EXERCISE to strengthen the muscles of the spine.

<u>Proper precautions on how to lift and good postural habits are essential for all people whether they have a scoliosis or a straight spine, to protect their spine from injury.</u>

CHAPTER EIGHT

Reasoning for the development and design of the home " SPINAL ACTIVE FLEXION EXERCISES" in short (S.A.F.E.)

Somebody said "that all the advances of the human race were made by somebody making an observation about something and somebody else adding to that observation. "

For example someone observed that wood floats on water, others added to that observation and today we have the huge ships we use.

Somebody invented the wheel and by continually somebody adding something to the invention of the wheel, today we have the cars and everything else that has wheels.

A young doctor observed that the women in a particular hospital were dying after they gave birth in that hospital while other women that were having their babies delivered at home by a midwife were not dying, not even getting sick.

On further observation he noticed that the same

doctors that they were doing autopsies on the dead mothers, they were examining the new mothers to be without washing their hands transferring the germs from the dead mothers to the new mothers to be and that's why the new mothers were dying from infections.

When he asked all the doctors to wash their hands when leaving the autopsy room and just before entering the room of the new mothers to be, the deaths of the new mothers stopped.

That's why today there is a lot of hand washing and sterilization to avoid infections and deaths during medical exams and operations.

The same goes for all the other inventions we have today that make our lives easier.

In 1865 William ADAMS was the first to describe " the forward bending test " for scoliosis, and all doctors use this test to diagnose the functional or structural scoliosis.

A functional scoliosis is the one that when the patient bends forward the spine straightens out and it is symmetrical at the thoracic level,
and with the structural scoliosis when the patient bends forward the abnormal curvature of the spine it is still noticeable but tries to straighten somewhat.

William Adams made a very good observation about the abnormal curve of the spine called scoliosis but nobody added anything to that observation or took advantage of that observation up to now.

Based on Williams Adams observation I designed specific exercises for the spine so that by bending and exercising the spine for long periods of time will make the muscles of the spine stronger , flexible and keep it almost straight.

Anybody who wants to correct the scoliotic spine they must first have the full co-operation of the patient to do the exercises everyday religiously , otherwise

NO TREATMENT OR EXERCISE

will correct the abnormal curvature if the patient keeps doing the bad habits that caused the abnormal curve in the first place.

FOR PEOPLE THAT ARE REALLY SERIOUS TO STOP THE PROGRESSION OF THE ABNORMAL SPINAL CURVE (THE SCOLIOSIS) AND EVEN REVERSE IT BACK TO ALMOST NORMAL

THEY SHOULD DO 3 THINGS

.1) STOP THE THINGS YOU ARE DOING TO CAUSE THE SCOLIOSIS, I.E. POOR POSTURE, POOR SITTING HABITS AT HOME, AT SCHOOL, PLAYING VIDEO GAMES AND SLOUCHING WHILE IN BAD SITTING POSITIONS WATCHING TELEVISION AND CARRYING HEAVY OBJECTS BACK PACKS AND EVEN BABIES ON ONE SIDE OF YOUR BODY.

2) SIT UPRIGHT ON THE CHAIR AT HOME, AT SCHOOL, WATCHING TV OR ON THE COMPUTER. AND STOP LIFTING AND HOLDING BABIES. IF YOU LOVE BABIES PLAY WITH THEM ON THE FLOOR, EVEN CRAWL AROUND WITH THE BABIES AND THAT'S GOOD FOR YOUR SPINE. SIT TALL, WALK TALL, FEEL TALL AND EXERCISE. EXERCISING WILL KEEP YOU HEALTHY AND HAVE A GOOD POSTURE.

3) DO THE RIGHT EXERCISES TO STRETCH, MOBILIZE YOUR SPINE AND STRENGTHEN YOUR SPINAL MUSCLES AND THAT WILL HELP YOUR SCOLIOSIS, IT CAN EVEN REVERSE IT.

YOU HAVE TO DO ALL 3:

A) STOP THE BAD HABITS THAT ARE CAUSING SCOLIOSIS

B) GET GOOD HABITS THAT HELP YOUR SPINE STAY STRAIGHT

C) DO THE RIGHT EXERCISES S.A.F.E. I designed

RELIGIOUSLY EVERY DAY TO MAKE YOUR SPINE STRONGER, FLEXIBLE AND STOP THE PROGRESSION OF THE ABNORMAL CURVE.

IF YOU DO ONLY ONE WILL NOT HELP YOU MUCH.

I WILL DESCRIBE THE RIGHT EXERCISES

BUT YOU HAVE TO DO THE WORK FAITHFULLY DAILY,

NOBODY ELSE CAN DO IT FOR YOU.

I THINK IT IS ABOUT TIME TO RECOGNIZE THAT SCOLIOSIS IS A PREVENTABLE DISEASE AND

SHIFT THE RESPONSIBILITY TO PREVENT AND CORRECT THE ABNORMAL CURVE TO THE PATIENT AND THEIR PARENTS,

BY GIVING THE PATIENT THE NECESSARY TOOLS, WHICH IN THIS CASE IS THE SPINAL EXERCISES, TO DO IT, IN THE PRIVACY OF THEIR HOME IN THEIR OWN BED!

NOBODY ELSE CAN DO IT FOR THEM.

AND UNFORTUNATELY NOBODY WILL EVER INVENT THE MAGIC PILL TO CORRECT THE SPINAL ABNORMAL CURVES!!!

IT IS A STRUCTURAL PROBLEM AND ONLY WITH EXERCISES CAN BE PREVENTED AND TREATED SUCCESSFULLY IN THE EARLY STAGES.

IF LEFT UNTREATED AND BECOMES SEVERE SCOLIOSIS THEY WILL END UP WITH CORRECTIVE SURGERY AND RODS IN THEIR SPINE!

FOR HOW LONG YOU HAVE TO DO THE EXERCISES?

I SAY FOREVER OR AT LEAST UNTIL

ADULTHOOD FOR THE GOOD OF YOUR SPINE AND YOUR HEALTH.

THE BEST TIME TO START EXERCISING IS YESTERDAY

BUT SINCE YESTERDAY IS GONE START AS SOON AS POSSIBLE OR RIGHT AFTER THE FIRST X RAY AND YOU WERE TOLD TO WAIT AND SEE FOR THE NEXT X RAY.

IF YOU CONTINUE WITH YOUR OLD BAD HABITS YOUR SCOLIOSIS WILL GET WORSE AND MIGHT NEED SURGERY IN THE FUTURE.

INSTEAD OF WAITING TO SEE WHAT HAPPENS TILL THE NEXT X RAY,

DO THESE EXERCISES AND AVOID YOUR OLD BAD SITTING HABITS, SIT STRAIGHT AT HOME, AT SCHOOL AND EVERYWHERE, DO NOT Slouch WHEN YOU WATCH TV OR PLAY VIDEO GAMES.

SIT TALL, WALK TALL, HAVE A GOOD POSTURE. AND THE NEXT TIME THEY TAKE YOUR X RAY YOU MIGHT BE SURPRISED TO SEE SOME IMPROVEMENT.

THE REASON I CHOSE THESE EXERCISES IS
THAT EVERY SPINE WITH SCOLIOSIS TRIES TO CORRECT ITSELF WHEN YOU BEND FORWARD (ADAMS TEST) SO IF YOU BEND YOUR SPINE OVER AND OVER ,YOUR SPINE WILL GET STRONGER AND STRAIGHTEN ITSELF TO A DEGREE.

WHEN I WAS DESIGNING THE SPINAL ACTIVE EXERCISES I PUT A LOT OF EMPHASIS ON THE LUMBAR , SACRAL, PELVIS AND HIP JOINTS, BECAUSE THAT'S WHERE MOST OF THE SCOLIOSIS START

AND BY MOBILIZING AND CORRECTING THOSE JOINTS WILL AFFECT THE SPINAL CURVES ABOVE.
YOU HAVE TO FIX THE FOUNDATION OF THE SPINE FIRST AND BY DOING SO THE SPINE WILL CORRECT ITSELF.. WHEN THE MUSCLES ARE STRONGER AND THE SPINAL JOINTS, HIP AND PELVIS ARE MOBILIZED .
OF COURSE YOU HAVE TO BE SURE THAT THERE IS NO PROBLEM WITH THE LEG LENGTHS , WITH THE LEGS BEING
THE REAL FOUNDATION OF THE SPINE AND THE WHOLE BODY.

I chose not to use the standing forward bending exercise, the Adams test, although it is a good exercise and will help the scoliotic spine and I designed the exercises to use the forward flexion of the spine while lying down face up taking away the gravity factor which is present when you stand and bend forward. Besides bending forward while standing over and over again might cause some strain on the low back and might be some other factors that the standing forward flexion is contraindicated, like some abnormality in the vertebral bones, like an undiagnosed fracture spondylolisthesis. , or spondylolysis.

If there are no contraindications and all the vertebrae have no break in the pars interarticularis (spondylolysis) or spondylolisthesis,

the Adam's forward bend is a good exercise to do several times a day.

MOST OF THE EXERCISES ARE DONE

LYING FACE UP SO THAT YOU CAN EASILY DO THE EXERCISES EVERY MORNING RIGHT AFTER YOU WAKE UP,, NOON AND AFTERNOON WITHOUT

STRAINING YOURSELF.

ALL EXERCISES SHOULD BE DONE ON AN EMPTY STOMACH AND GO EASY AT THE BEGINNING WITHOUT STRAINING YOURSELF UNTIL YOUR SPINE GETS STRONGER AND MORE FLEXIBLE WITH THE DAILY SPINAL STRETCHING.

AS YOUR SPINAL MUSCLES ARE GETTING STRONGER YOU INCREASE THE REPETITION OF THE EXERCISES TO HAVE BETTER RESULTS SOONER!

CHAPTER NINE

DESCRIPTIONS OF THE HOME S.A.F.E. EXERCISES AND HERE ARE THE HOME EXERCISES WHICH I DESIGNED AND I CALL S.A.F.E. (SPINAL ACTIVE FLEXION EXERCISES)

1) spinal stretch by extending your arms above your head and your legs extended with feet together touching the mattress pushing them down as much as possible

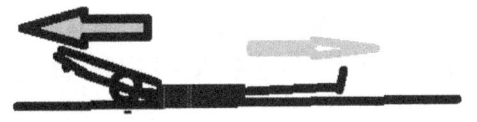

EXTEND YOUR HANDS ABOVE YOUR HEAD TRYING TO REACH AS FAR AS YOU CAN AND SIMULTANEOUSLY
WITH YOUR FEET TOGETHER TOUCHING THE MATTRESS STRETCH THEM DOWN AS FAR AS YOU CAN

THIS IS A SPINAL STRETCH EXERCISE
FEEL THE SPINAL STRETCH

LIE FACE UP ON A FIRM MATTRESS WITH A SMALL PILLOW UNDER YOUR HEAD OR YOU CAN DO THESE EXERCISES IN YOUR OWN BED RIGHT AFTER YOU WAKE UP IN THE MORNING.

EXTEND BOTH YOUR FEET TOGETHER

TOUCHING THE MATTRESS

AND EXTEND YOUR HANDS ABOVE YOUR HEAD AS FAR AS YOU CAN WITH YOUR RIGHT HAND HOLDING YOU LEFT WRIST

STRETCH YOUR HANDS UP

AND YOUR FEET DOWN TRYING TO EXTEND YOUR SPINE AS MUCH AS POSSIBLE

WHILE TAKING A DEEP BREATH EXPANDING YOUR CHEST AS MUCH AS POSSIBLE
'FEEL THE STRETCH OF YOUR SPINE

HOLD IT FOR THE COUNT OF THREE'

AND THEN EXHALE SLOWLY

REPEAT IT 5 TIMES. OR MORE

THIS IS A STRETCHING EXERCISE OF YOUR SPINE

THEN EXERCISE

2) EXERCISE STRETCHING YOUR CHEST AND SHOULDER BLADES

LYING FACE UP WITH FEET EXTENDED

INTERLOCK YOUR FINGERS

AND PLACE YOUR HANDS UNDER YOUR HEAD

AND YOUR ELBOWS TOUCHING THE MATTRESS.

THEN BRING YOUR ELBOWS TOWARDS YOUR FACE AND THEN BACK PRESSING ON THE MATTRESS.

EXERCISE STRETCHING YOUR CHEST AND SHOULDER
LYING FACE UP WITH FEET EXTENDED
INTERLOCK YOUR FINGERS AND PLACE YOUR HANDS UNDER YOUR HEAD AND YOUR ELBOWS TOUCHING THE MATTRESS.

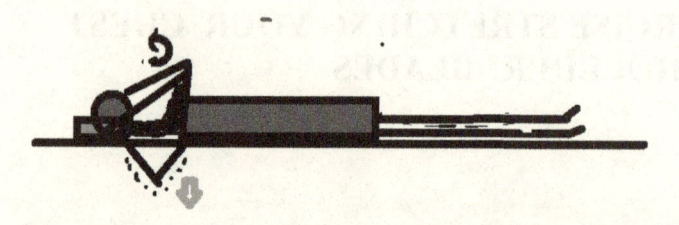

INTERLOCK YOUR FINGERS AND PLACE YOUR HANDS UNDER YOUR HEAD AND YOUR ELBOWS TOUCHING THE MATTRESS.
THEN
BRING YOUR ELBOWS TOWARDS YOUR FACE AND THEN BACK PRESSING ON THE MATTRESS.

REPEAT THIS EXERCISE 5-10 TIMES .

REST BY TAKING A FEW DEEP BREATHS EXPANDING YOUR CHEST AS MUCH AS POSSIBLE AND THEN EXHALING SLOWLY

THIS IS A GOOD STRETCHING EXERCISE FOR YOUR SHOULDER BLADES AND UPPER BACK MUSCLES

THE ABOVE EXERCISES INCREASE THE MOBILITY OF YOUR CHEST , NECK AND UPPER BACK STRENGTHENING THE MUSCLES OF YOUR BACK , SHOULDER

BLADES AND RIBS.

3) SPINAL STRETCH

RAISING YOUR HEAD TOWARDS YOUR CHEST

WHILE SUPPORTING YOUR HEAD WITH YOUR HANDS

FROM THE SAME POSITION,

LYING FACE UP,

YOUR FEET EXTENDED

AND WITH YOUR INTERLOCKED FINGERS SUPPORTING YOUR HEAD,

RAISE YOUR HEAD TOWARDS YOUR CHEST AS FAR AS YOU CAN

WITHOUT STRAINING YOUR SELF

AND THEN LOWER IT GENTLY TO THE PILLOW

AND PRESS YOUR HEAD ON THE PILLOW

FEELING THE STRETCH OF YOUR SPINE

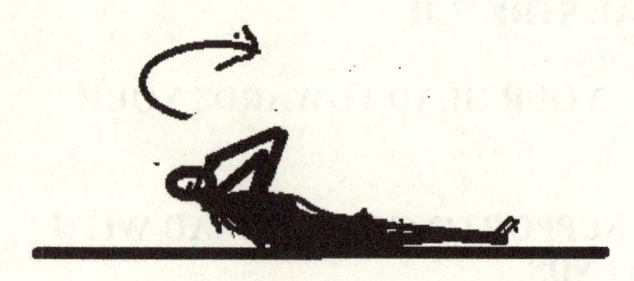

RAISE YOUR HEAD TO YOUR CHEST AS MUCH AS YOU CAN WITHOUT STRAINING YOURSELF,
AND THEN LET YOUR HEAD AND HANDS GENTLY DOWN TO THE MATTRESS.

REPEAT 5-10 TIMES AND KEEP INCREASING THEM EVERY WEEK

THIS EXERCISE STRETCHES YOUR WHOLE SPINE

N.B....IF YOU FIND IT DIFFICULT TO DO THIS EXERCISE WITH YOUR HANDS UNDER YOUR HEAD,
YOU CAN PLACE YOUR HANDS FLAT ON YOUR LOWER ABDOMEN AND DO THIS EXERCISE UNTIL YOU ARE STRONGER AND YOU CAN DO IT WITH YOUR HANDS SUPPORTING YOUR HEAD.

4) KNEE TO CHEST

AND RAISE YOUR HEAD TOWARDS YOUR KNEE

LYING FACE UP,

INTERLOCKED FINGERS UNDER YOUR HEAD

AND LEGS EXTENDED FEET TOGETHER ON THE MATTRESS

A) BEND YOUR RIGHT KNEE

AND BRING IT TOWARDS YOUR CHEST

THEN RAISE YOUR HEAD TOWARDS YOUR BEND KNEE

WITHOUT STRAINING YOURSELF

LYING FACE UP,
INTERLOCKED FINGERS
UNDER YOUR HEAD AND LEGS
EXTENDED FEET TOGETHER
ON THE MATTRESS

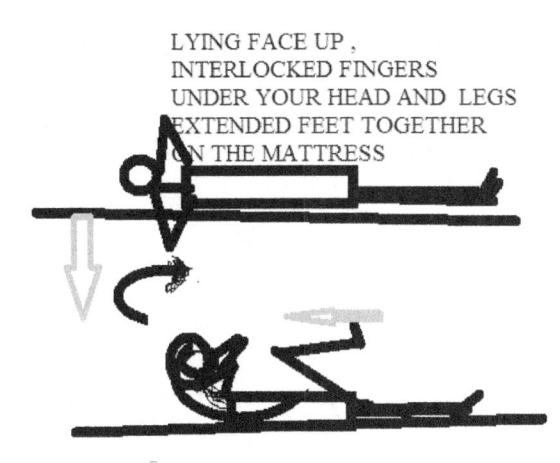

BEND YOUR RIGHT KNEE AND BRING IT TOWARDS YOUR CHEST
THEN RAISE YOUR HEAD TOWARDS YOUR BEND KNEE
WITHOUT STRAINING YOURSELF

AND HOLD FOR THE COUNT OF TWO

LOWER YOU'RE HEAD GENTLY ON THE MATTRESS

IN ADDITION, EXTEND YOUR KNEE.

B) REPEAT THE SAME EXERCISE WITH LEFT KNEE

THEN BEND YOUR LEFT KNEE

AND BRING IT TOWARDS YOUR CHEST

THEN RAISE YOUR HEAD TOWARDS YOUR KNEE

WITHOUT STRAINING YOURSELF,

HOLD THIS POSITION FOR THE COUNT OF TWO

AND THEN LOWER YOUR HEAD GENTLY TO THE MATTRESS

IN ADDITION, EXTEND YOUR KNEE.

5) BOTH KNEES TO CHEST

AND RAISING YOUR HEAD TOWARDS YOUR KNEES

LYING FACE UP,

INTERLOCKED FINGERS UNDER YOUR HEAD

BEND YOUR KNEES

AND BRING THEM TO YOUR CHEST

AS CLOSE AS POSSIBLE

WITHOUT STRAINING G YOURSELF

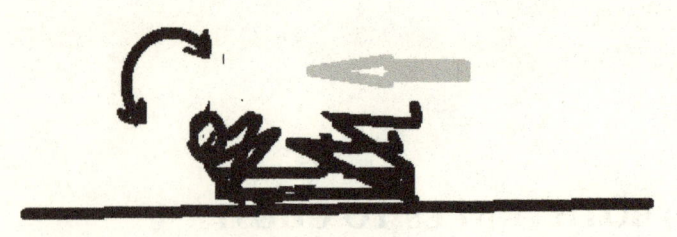

LYING FACE UP , INTERLOCKED FINGERS
UNDER YOUR HEAD
BEND YOUR KNEES AND BRING THEM TO
YOUR CHEST AS CLOSE AS POSSIBLE WITHOUT
STRAINING G YOURSELF
AND RAISE YOUR HEAD TOWARDS YOUR
KNEES

AND RAISE YOUR HEAD TOWARDS YOUR KNEES

HOLD FOR THE COUNT OF TWO

AND LOWER YOUR HEAD GENTLY TO THE MATTRESS

AND YOUR BENT KNEES TO THE MATTRESS

REPEAT THIS EXERCISE 5 TIMES

REST BY TAKING A DEEP BREATH

AND EXHALING SLOWLY

DEEP BREATHING IS VERY IMPORTANT EXERCISE AS IT EXPANDS YOUR CHEST RIBS FORCING THEM TO RETURN TO THEIR NORMAL PLACE!!!

6) SPINAL ACTIVE FLEXION EXERCISE

 **BENT KNEE TO SIDE
AND RAISING YOUR HEAD**

LYING FACE UP,

YOUR INTERLOCKED FINGERS UNDER YOUR HEAD

AND YOUR KNEES BENT WITH FEET FIRMLY FLAT ON THE MATTRESS

A) LET YOUR BENT RIGHT KNEE SLIDE TO YOUR RIGHT SIDE TOUCHING THE MATTRESS

THEN RAISE YOUR HEAD TOWARDS YOUR CHEST

WITHOUT STRAINING YOURSELF

HOLD TO THE COUNT OF TWO

THEN LOWER YOUR HEAD GENTLY TO THE MATTRESS

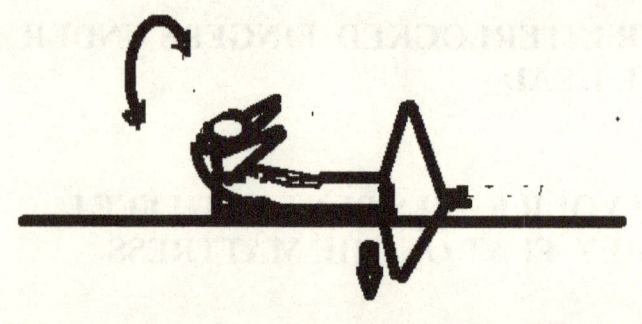

LET YOUR BENT RIGHT KNEE SLIDE TO YOUR
RIGHT SIDE TOUCHING THE MATTRESS
THEN RAISE YOUR HEAD TOWARDS YOUR CHEST
WITHOUT STRAINING YOURSELF
HOLD TO THE COUNT OF TWO
THEN LOWER YOUR HEAD GENTLY TO THE
MATTRESS AND YOUR RIGHT KNEE BACK UP TO
TOUCH THE LEFT KNEE

AND YOUR RIGHT KNEE BACK UP TO TOUCH THE LEFT KNEE

B) LET YOUR BENT LEFT KNEE SLIDE TO YOUR LEFT SIDE TO TOUCH THE MATTRESS

THEN RAISE YOUR HEAD TOWARDS YOUR CHEST

WITHOUT STRAINING YOUR SELF ,

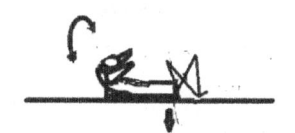

LET YOUR BENT RIGHT KNEE SLIDE TO YOUR
RIGHT SIDE TOUCHING THE MATTRESS
THEN RAISE YOUR HEAD TOWARDS YOUR CHEST
WITHOUT STRAINING YOURSELF
HOLD TO THE COUNT OF TWO
THEN LOWER YOUR HEAD GENTLY TO THE
MATTRESS AND YOUR RIGHT KNEE BACK UP TO
TOUCH THE LEFT KNEE

HOLD FOR THE COUNT OF TWO

THEN LOWER YOUR HEAD

GENTLY TO THE MATTRESS
AND YOUR LEFT KNEE BACK UP TO THE OTHER KNEE

REPEAT THIS EXERCISE 5 TIMES EACH KNEE

THIS EXERCISE IS VERY GOOD TO MOBILIZE YOUR HIPS, PELVIC JOINTS AND THE JOINTS OF YOUR WHOLE SPINE

EVERY WEEK YOU INCREASE THEM UNTIL YOU REACH 20-30

WITHOUT STRAINING YOURSELF.

7) RAISING YOUR LOW BACK TOWARDS THE CEILING

LYING DOWN FACE UP WITH YOUR KNEES BENT

AND YOUR HANDS UNDER YOUR HEAD

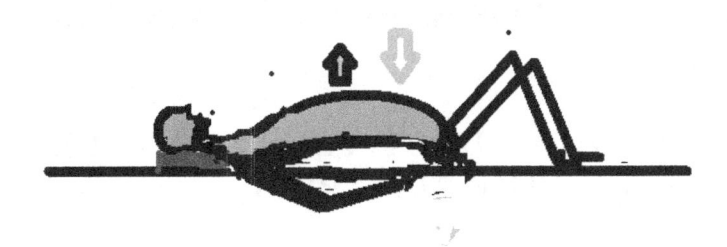

LYING DOWN FACE UP WITH YOUR KNEES BENT
AND YOUR HANDS ON THE SIDE BESIDES YOUR LOW BACK
RAISE YOUR LOW BACK TOWARDS THE CEILING AND THEN DOWN,
UP AND DOWN FOR 5-10 TIMES OR MORE WITHOUT YOUR LOW BACK TOUCHING THE MATTRESS
AND THEN LOWER YOUR LOW BACK GENTLY TO THE MATTRESS.

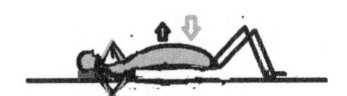

LYING DOWN FACE UP WITH YOUR KNEES BENT
AND YOUR INTELACED HANDS UNDER YOUR HEAD
RAISE YOUR LOW BACK TOWARDS THE CEILING AND THEN DOWN,
UP AND DOWN FOR 5-10 TIMES OR MORE WITHOUT YOUR LOW BACK TOUCHING THE MATTRESS
AND THEN LOWER YOUR LOW BACK GENTLY TO THE MATTRESS.

RAISE YOUR LOW BACK TOWARDS THE CEILING

AND THEN DOWN, UP AND DOWN FOR 5-10 TIMES

OR MORE WITHOUT YOUR LOW BACK TOUCHING THE MATTRESS

THEN LOWER YOUR LOW BACK GENTLY TO THE MATTRESS.

REST BY TAKING A BREATH OR TWO

REPEAT THIS EXERCISE 10 TIMES

AND EVERY WEEK YOU INCREASE THEM UNTIL YOU REACH 20-30

WITHOUT STRAINING YOURSELF.

8) SPINAL ACTIVE FLEXION EXERCISES

KNEE TO CHEST EXERCISE

LYING FACE UP WITH YOUR KNEES BENT
AND YOUR HANDS ON YOUR SIDE

A) DRAW YOUR RIGHT KNEE TO YOUR CHEST

GRAB IT WITH BOTH HANDS AND PRESS IT ON YOUR CHEST,

AND RAISE YOUR HEAD TOWARDS YOUR KNEE

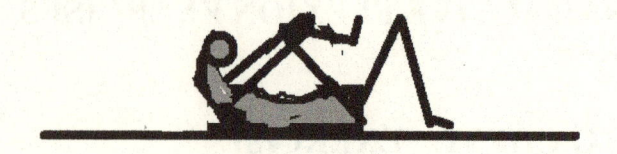

A) DRAW YOUR RIGHT KNEE TO YOUR CHEST
GRAB IT WITH BOTH HANDS AND PRESS IT ON YOUR CHEST,
AND RAISE YOUR HEAD TOWARDS YOUR KNEE

HOLD IT FOR THE COUNT OF TWO
THEN RETURN IT TO ITS ORIGINAL BENT POSITION.

HOLD IT FOR THE COUNT OF TWO

THEN RETURN IT TO ITS ORIGINAL BENT POSITION

. B) THEN FROM THE SAME POSITION

DRAW YOUR LEFT KNEE TO YOUR CHEST

GRASP IT WITH BOTH HANDS AND PRESS IT ON YOUR CHEST

AND RAISE YOUR HEAD TOWARDS YOUR KNEE

.HOLD IT FOR THE COUNT OF TWO

THEN RETURN IT TO ITS ORIGINAL BENT POSITION.

REPEAT THIS EXERCISE 5-10 TIMES ON EACH KNEE THEN REST FOR 2-3 MINUTES

9) KNEES TO CHEST EXERCISES

AND RAISE YOUR HEAD TOWARDS YOUR BENT KNEES

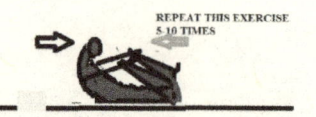

REPEAT THIS EXERCISE
5-10 TIMES

WITH YOUR KNEES BENT DRAW BOTH KNEES TO YOUR CHEST,
GRAB YOUR KNEES WITH BOTH HANDS DRAWING THE KNEES AS NEAR
TO THE CHEST AS POSSIBLE,
AND THEN RAISE YOUR HEAD TOWARDS YOUR KNEES

WITHOUT STRAINING YOURSELF

HOLD IT FOR THE COUNT OF TWO

THEN LOWER YOUR HEAD GENTLY TO THE MATTRESS
AND YOUR FEET TO THE MATTRESS

FROM THE SAME POSITION

LYING FACE UP

WITH YOUR KNEES BENT

DRAW BOTH KNEES TO YOUR CHEST,

GRAB YOUR KNEES WITH BOTH HANDS

DRAWING THE KNEES AS NEAR TO THE CHEST AS POSSIBLE.

AND THEN RAISE YOUR HEAD TOWARDS YOUR KNEES

WITHOUT STRAINING YOURSELF

HOLD IT FOR THE COUNT OF TWO

THEN LOWER YOUR HEAD GENTLY TO THE MATTRESS

AND YOUR FEET TO THE MATTRESS

DO THIS EXERCISE 5-10 TIMES

WITHOUT STRAINING YOURSELF

10) KNEES TO CHEST ROCKING EXERCISE

Knees to chest rocking exercises : this is the most important exercise to increase the flexibility of your spine.

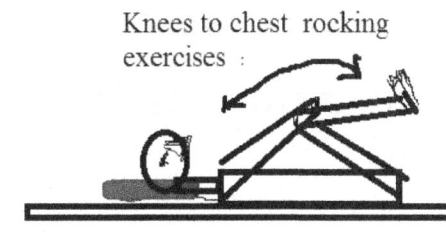

grab your right knee with your right hand and your left knee with your left hand and bring your knees to your chest and with a rocking motion rock your pelvis back and forth

LYING FACE UP WITH YOUR KNEES BENT

AND YOUR HANDS ON YOUR SIDE

BRING YOUR BENT KNEES TOWARDS YOUR CHEST

GRASP YOUR RIGHT KNEE WITH YOUR RIGHT HAND

AND YOUR LEFT KNEE WITH YOUR LEFT

HAND

AND PRESS THEM ON YOUR CHEST,

WHILE HOLDING YOUR KNEES ABOUT 6 INCHES APART WITH YOUR HANDS

WITH A ROCKING MOVE

ROCK YOUR PELVIS BACK AND FORTH

BY BRING YOUR KNEES TO YOUR CHEST

AND BACK WITHOUT YOUR FEET TOUCHING THE MATTRESS

REPEAT THIS EXERCISE 10-20 TIMES

WITHOUT STRAINING YOUR SELF

AND INCREASE EVERY WEEK BY 5 MORE TIMES

UNTIL YOU CAN EASILY DO 100.

REST FOR A FEW SECONDS
OR MORE DEPENDING HOW YOU FEEL

BY TAKING DEEP BREATHS

AND EXHALING SLOWLY.

REMEMBER NOT TO OVERDO IT WITH
THE EXERCISES.

START SLOWLY WITH A FEW AND
INCREASING THEM

AS YOU GET STRONGER

THIS IS A VERY IMPORTANT EXERCISE,
AND THIS IS THE MAXIMUM BEND
FORWARD THAT MIMICS THE ADAMS
TEST STRETCHING THE SPINE TO ITS
MAXIMUM WITHOUT GRAVITY.

THIS EXERCISE MOBILIZES ALL JOINTS
OF THE SPINE, HIP AND PELVIS JOINTS
AND CHEST AND SHOULDER JOINTS

11) SPINAL STRETCH MIMICKING

THE BICYCLES PEDALING MOVES

11) SPINAL STRETCH MIMICKING THE BICYCLES MOVES

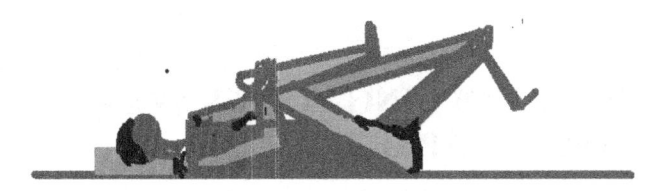

WHILE HOLDING YOUR KNEES ABOUT 6 INCHES APART WITH YOUR HANDS
BRING YOUR LEFT KNEE UP TOWARDS YOUR CHEST
AND SIMULTANEOUSLY PUSH YOUR RIGHT KNEE DOWN TOWARDS THE MATTRESS WITHOUT TOUCHING THE MATTRESS
WHILE YOU STILL HOLD YOUR KNEES
AND KEEP MOVING ONE KNEE UP AND THE OTHER DOWN MIMICKING THE PEDALING OF A BICYCLE

LYING FACE UP WITH YOUR KNEES BENT

AND YOUR HANDS BY YOUR SIDE

BRING YOUR BENT KNEES TOWARDS YOUR CHEST

GRASP YOUR RIGHT KNEE WITH YOUR RIGHT HAND

AND YOUR LEFT KNEE WITH YOUR LEFT HAND

AND WHILE HOLDING YOUR KNEES ABOUT 6 INCHES APART

WITH YOUR HANDS

BRING YOUR LEFT KNEE UP TOWARDS YOUR CHEST

AND SIMULTANEOUSLY PUSH YOUR RIGHT KNEE

DOWN TOWARDS THE MATTRESS WITHOUT TOUCHING THE MATTRESS

WHILE YOU STILL HOLD YOUR KNEES

AND KEEP MOVING ONE KNEE UP

AND THE OTHER DOWN

MIMICKING THE PEDALING OF A BICYCLE

KEEP DOING IT FOR THE COUNT OF FIFTY ,

WHICH IS ABOUT A MINUTE,

BUT DO NOT EXERT YOURSELF.

12) SPINAL STRETCH

WHILE LYING DOWN FACE UP.

EXTEND YOUR HANDS ABOVE YOUR

HEAD

TRYING TO REACH AS FAR AS YOU CAN

AND SIMULTANEOUSLY WITH YOUR FEET TOGETHER TOUCHING THE MATTRESS

STRETCH THEM DOWN AS FAR AS YOU CAN

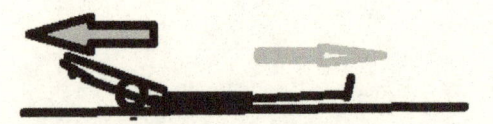

EXTEND YOUR HANDS ABOVE YOUR HEAD TRYING TO REACH AS FAR AS YOU CAN
AND SIMULTANEOUSLY
WITH YOUR FEET TOGETHER TOUCHING THE MATTRESS STRETCH THEM DOWN AS FAR AS YOU CAN

THIS IS A SPINAL STRETCH EXERCISE
FEEL THE SPINAL STRETCH

TAKE A DEEP BREATH

EXPANDING YOUR CHEST AS MUCH AS POSSIBLE

THIS IS A SPINAL STRETCH EXERCISE

FEEL THE SPINAL STRETCH

EXHALE SLOWLY,

REPEAT 5 TIMES OR MORE

N.B. If there are no contraindications you can ALSO do the Adams forward flexion exercise during the day.

13) ADAMS BEND FORWARDS TEST EXERCISE

START WITH THE STANDING POSITION,

FEET AND KNEES TOGETHER,

BEND FORWARD TRYING TO REACH YOUR TOES WITH THE FINGERS OF YOUR HANDS

ADAMS BEND FORWARDS TEST EXERCISE

START WITH THE STANDING POSITION, FEET AND KNEES TOGETHER, BEND FORWARD TRYING TO REACH YOUR TOES WITH THE FINGERS OF YOUR HANDS

THIS EXERCISE STRETCHES YOUR WHOLE SPINE AND THE SPINE STRAIGHTENS IN FUNCTIONAL SCOLIOSIS, AND TRIES TO STRAIGHTEN IN STRUCTURAL SCOLIOSIS

THIS EXERCISE STRETCHES YOUR WHOLE SPINE

AND THE SPINE STRAIGHTENS IN FUNCTIONAL SCOLIOSIS.

AND TRIES TO STRAIGHTEN IN STRUCTURAL SCOLIOSIS.

14) MODIFIED ADAMS FORWARD BEND TEST EXERCISE

START WITH THE STANDING POSITION

BUT YOUR FEET ARE PLACED 12-18 INCHES APART

BEND FORWARDS

AND TOUCH YOUR LEFT FOOT WITH YOUR RIGHT HAND FINGERS

WHILE YOUR LEFT HAND IS AT THE BACK OF YOUR LOW BACK

START WITH THE STANDING POSITION BUT
YOUR FEET ARE PLACED 12-18 INCHES APART
BEND FORWARDS AND TOUCH YOUR LEFT
FOOT WITH YOUR RIGHT HAND FINGERS
WHILE YOUR LEFT HAND RESTS ON THE BACK
OF YOUR LOW BACK

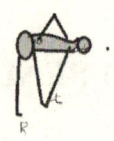

YOU COME UP TO STRAIGHT POSITION

AND THEN BEND FORWARDS AND TOUCH YOUR RIGHT FOOT

WITH YOUR LEFT HAND FINGERS

NB. IF YOU HAVE A NOTICEABLE RIB HUMP

ON YOUR RIGHT SIDE,

THEN DO TWICE AS MANY BENDS

WITH YOUR RIGHT HAND TO YOUR LEFT FOOT

AND VICE VERSA.

THIS IS DONE BECAUSE WHEN YOU BRING YOUR RIGHT HAND (THE SIDE OF YOUR HUMP) TO YOUR LEFT FOOT THE BENDING STRETCH DRAWS FORWARD YOUR HUMP AND CORRECTS YOUR RIB CAGE

AND WITH TIME IT SHOULD BRING IT BACK TO NORMAL ,THAT'S WHY YOU DO THE BENDS TWICE AS MUCH ON THE SIDE

OF HUMP.

DO THESE EXERCISES 3 TIMES A DAY

UNLESS YOU ARE SICK OR HAVE FEVER IN WHICH CASE YOU DO NOT DO ANY EXERCISES

THESE ARE THE MAIN EXERCISES BASED ON THE ADAMS BEND FORWARD TEST, THAT WILL HELP YOUR SCOLIOSIS

BUT YOU HAVE TO DO THEM EVERY DAY RELIGIOUSLY

3 TIMES A DAY, MORNING WHEN YOU WAKE UP AND TWICE IN THE AFTERNOON

AS WITH ANY OTHER EXERCISES , YOU EXERCISE ON AN EMPTY STOMACH.

AND TAKE IT EASY AT THE BEGINNING UNTIL YOUR BODY GETS STRONGER, FLEXIBLE AND YOU HAVE MORE ENDURANCE

OTHER EXERCISES THAT WILL HELP YOU STRAIGHTEN OUT YOUR SPINE ARE

THE MONKEY BAR WHICH I HIGHLY RECOMMEND

YOU USE ANY TIME YOU HAVE THE CHANCE

.MAYBE EVERYDAY

15) USE A MONKEY BAR TO EXERCISE.

WHICH IS VERY GOOD FOR STRETCHING YOUR SPINE

EXERCISING ON THE MONKEY BAR

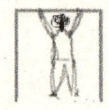

GRAB THE MONKEY BAR WITH BOTH HANDS

AND LET YOUR BODY SWING BACK AND FORTH A FEW TIMES,

AND YOU CAN DO SOME CHIN UPS IF

YOU WANT

.REPEAT IT OFTEN WITHOUT STRAINING YOURSELF.

THIS EXERCISE STRETCHES YOUR SPINE NATURALLY WITH YOUR OWN BODY. WEIGHT...

BESIDES MONKEYS DO IT ALL THE TIME

AND THEY NEVER GET SCOLIOSIS.

16) SWIMMING IS AN EXCELLENT EXERCISE FOR SCOLIOSIS.

TRY TO SWIM 1-2 TIMES A WEEK IF YOU CAN.

I HIGHLY RECOMMEND IT.

SWIMMING EXERCISES ALL THE MUSCLES OF THE BODY

AND I HIGHLY RECOMMEND IT.

BESIDES FISHES THAT SWIM ALL THE TIME,

DO NOT GET SCOLIOSIS.

17) WALKING IS AN EXCELLENT EXERCISE

MAKE IT A HABIT TO WALK DAILY WITHOUT SLOUCHING.

BE PROUD OF YOUR BODY AND YOUR POSTURE!

NB: THE s.a.f.e. EXERCISES ARE GOOD FOR ANYONE THAT HAS A SPINE BUT NOT FOR PEOPLE WITH TRAUMA, PATHOLOGY OR HAD SURGERY AND RODS.

IT IS VERY GOOD FOR PEOPLE WITH FUNCTIONAL SCOLIOSIS BUT IT WILL HELP ONLY IF PEOPLE WITH SCOLIOSIS CHANGE THEIR DAILY BAD POSTURAL HABITS AVOID BAD SITTING HABITS AND THEY SHOULD SIT STRAIGHT ON A CHAIR AT HOME AT SCHOOL, AND AVOID SLOUCHING, WHEN THEY WATCH TV OR PLAY VIDEO GAMES AND NEVER CARY HEAVY OBJECTS ON ONE SIDE OF THEIR BODY, SUCH AS HEAVY BACK PACKS ,OR BABIES............

………..REMEMBER, PEOPLE THAT EXERCISE DAILY HAVE GOOD POSTURE, GOOD HEALTH .A STRONG HEALTHY AND FLEXIBLE SPINE , NO ABNORMAL SPINAL CURVES.

AND NEVER GET SCOLIOSIS.....

I NEVER SAW ANY BODY BUILDER OR ANY OTHER ATHLETE THAT EXERCISES DAILY WITH SCOLIOSIS.

THE SOLUTION TO THIS PREVENTABLE CONDITION CALLED SCOLIOSIS IS SIMPLY ,EXERCISE DAILY AND NOT ANY MAGIC PILL INVENTED IN A LABORATORY...

I RECENTLY WATCHED A VIDEO ON YOU TUBE , MADE IN 2018 ,BY ARNOLD SCHWARZENEGGER AND SYLVESTER STALLONE EXERCISING, AND I THINK THEY ARE IN THEIR 70S, AND ARNOLD SAID " YOU HAVE TO EXERCISE DAILY".

LOOK AT THE SHAPE THEY ARE IN THEIR 70S?

DO YOU THINK THAT THOSE GUYS AND OTHERS THAT EXERCISE DAILY, COULD GET A SCOLIOSIS IN THEIR SPINE?

I DO NOT THINK SO.

Every day millions of people are doing some of the exercises i described above, or similar exercises, in the gyms , the military training their soldiers, at the beaches swimming, at schools and at home and they have strong healthy and flexible spines The only thing they have not realized is that these exercises helped them to avoid abnormal curves in their spines, scoliosis, kyphosis and lordosis. If the people that have scoliosis or any other abnormal curve, they were doing the right exercises , like the S.A.FE. I describe above they would also have a strong , healthy , flexible spine without any abnormal curves.
 EVEN after they got the abnormal curves, if they start exercising, their spine will get stronger , more flexible and with time they might reverse that abnormal curve, or at least stop the progression of that abnormal curve, if it is not that severe that requires surgery.

CHAPTER TEN

SUMMARY OF THE DAILY ROUTINE HOME EXERCISES " S.A.F.E". SPINAL FLEXION EXERCISES

IN SUMMARY THIS IS THE DAILY ROUTINE FOR THE S.A.F.E. EXERCISES.

START SLOWLY AND EASY AND AS YOU GET STRONGER AND MORE FLEXIBLE INCREASE THE TIMES YOU DO THESE EXERCISES.

NEVER OVER DO IT AND NEVER STRAIN

YOURSELF. BUILD UP YOUR ENDURANCE OVER TIME!

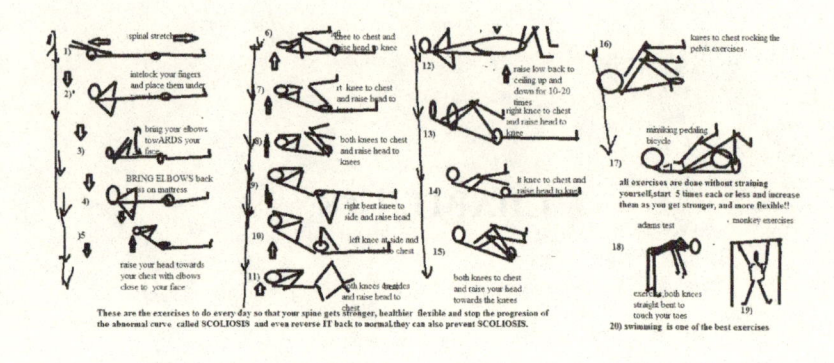

Regular exercise is important for children with scoliosis. It can help improve muscle strength and may help reduce the scoliosis and pain. Children with scoliosis can usually do most types of exercise safely. They only need to avoid certain activities such as lifting heavy objects or backpacks, and sit straight on the chair at home and school and avoid bad sitting or slouching when they watch TV or play video games. Poor posture and slouching should be avoided and never carry on the side of their body or shoulder.

Specific back exercises .such as the ones. I designed the S.A.F.E. exercises to help improve scoliosis by strengthening the back muscles and the flexibility of the spine.

Many children won't need any other treatment, provided that they exercise every day and avoid bad postural habits .Only a small number will end up having surgery if their scoliosis was advanced before starting the exercises.

Children and young people should also reduce the time they spend sitting for extended periods of time, watching TV, playing computer games and other prolong sitting activities.

GOOD LUCK TO ALL.

CHAPTER ELEVEN

EXPECTED RESULTS

The S.A.F.E. exercises are designed to give flexibility and strength to the spine as long as you do them daily.

To have good results you have to change your old habits of bad posture at home, at school and everywhere else.

If you do the exercises and keep doing what you have been doing that started the scoliosis, do not expect much, because you did not remove the CAUSE that started the scoliosis.

You might see some improvement but not as much as when you removed the cause, the bad posture habits. .

if you do the exercises daily three times a day and you removed the cause of the scoliosis, and if you are a girl you should stop lifting and carrying babies around , with these exercises along with some swimming exercises and monkey bar stretching exercises you should get good results in 2-3 months .

Even when you see some improvement you should keep doing the exercises daily for ever if you want to have a strong ,healthy, flexible spine, along with all the other benefits that come with a healthy spine. It will be taking you about

15 minutes times 3 a total of 45 minutes a day and the health benefits are good.

Of course you will be doing these exercises on an empty stomach and you should not exercise when you are sick with fever, infections or have pain.

I am not a believer of "NO PAIN NO GAIN." When there is pain it is a warning from your body to stop and you should always listen to your body.

CHAPTER TWELVE

RESEARCH:

Research is needed to identify the real multiple causes of the so called IDIOPATHIC SCOLIOSIS which is not idiopathic at all, they just did not recognize the cause.

To call it IDIOPATHIC and do nothing about it while we watch it to get worse ruining the lives of millions of youngsters I think it is not a good thing to do.

Or just believe in wild THEORIES that scoliosis is caused by the bones growing faster than the nerve trunks and the nerve trunks are pulling the bones into a scoliotic curve is absurd.

IF that was the case every time the surgeons fuse the spine and put rods to correct the scoliosis the nerve trunks would break leaving the patient with severe catastrophic neurological problems including paralysis, something which thankfully is not happening now.

Yes, I watched this video on YOU TUBE, a medical doctor holding a spine and pulling some strings to cause a scoliosis, claiming that was the real cause of IDIOPATHIC scoliosis according to the theory of some dr. Roth, that the bones are growing faster than the nerve trunks causing the spine into scoliosis.

Fortunately it is just a theory and I hope that not many doctors believe in that absurd theory, otherwise they will throw their hands up in the air and say there is nothing we can do about scoliosis and stop the search to reverse the abnormal curve.

WITH ALL THE ADVANCES IN TECHNOLOGY WE CAN EASILY IDENTIFY, AT LEAST WITH STATISTICS, WHAT'S CAUSING WHAT.

With the help of statistics we can know how many women had babies the natural way and what percentage of those babies develop infantile scoliosis. How many women had babies with the use of instrumentation and how many of those babies develop scoliosis, wry neck or had other health problems such as cerebral palsy etc.

How many women had their babies with cesarean section and how many of those babies develop scoliosis or other health problems? By analyzing those statistics we can see which method of delivering the babies is the most safe and causes less health problems to the mother and the baby, and if a woman has a difficult delivery instead of waiting and using instruments with the possibility to cause injuries to the new baby, let her have a cesarean section delivery instead.

How many kids are diagnoses with infantile scoliosis after a normal birth and under what conditions.

Give the mothers a questionnaire to fill out and see what is the common cause that causes the infantile scoliosis. Falls, injuries , or just bad positioning of the baby? when you recognize the common cause , name the scoliosis with that cause.
Such as POSITIONAL INFANTILE SCOLIOSIS when it is caused by bad positioning of the baby, or,
TRAUMATIC INFANTILE SCOLIOSIS when there is an injury or fall that caused the scoliosis, AND treat each condition accordingly.

With juvenile idiopathic scoliosis again try to find the cause and name the scoliosis accordingly. when we have a cause and a name it is easier to treat. Give the kids and their parents a questionnaire about their lifestyle and habits and see if there are common elements , in lifestyle or habits that cause the scoliosis and name it accordingly. BAD POSTURAL POSITIONS JUVENILE SCOLIOSIS, simply

POSTURAL JUVENILE SCOLIOSIS if it is due to daily bad postural positions, like slouching on the sofa watching television, studying, playing video games etc.

OR KIDS PLAYING WITH BABIES NAME IT 'BABYSITTING JUVENILE SCOLIOSIS ', if the kids baby-sit play with their siblings ,nephews or other babies for long periods of time.

Statistics can help identify the cause and when the cause is known it is not IDIOPATHIC ANYMORE, and by just eliminating the cause of the new named scoliosis and give them the right spinal stretching exercises the scoliosis will improve , even eliminated????.

Any research done it has to involve the youngsters that have the scoliosis to find the cause and eliminate whatever the cause is.

Any research done in the laboratory searching for genes or other causes without the involvement of those who already have the condition will not have any meaningful use in the treatment and correction of the abnormal curve. Looking at DNA markers for scoliosis and start performing surgeries on healthy youngsters that have the so

called DNA markers but no scoliosis yet, just with the laboratory theory that you will prevent future scoliosis it is absurd .
Spending billions of dollars for lab research for scoliosis without the involvement of real people that suffer from scoliosis, is a waste of money.
If , however you use the DNA markers to encourage the youngsters to exercise and prevent them from developing scoliosis, that would be acceptable and desirable.

Based on the observations of William Adams who Was the first to observe ,that a scoliotic spine tries to straighten out when bending forward(flexion of the spine) " the Adams forward bend test ," I devised specific spinal exercises for repeat flexion of the spine without the gravity, simply lying face up while doing the exercises,.

I hope that with these exercises which I call them SPINAL ACTIVE FLEXION EXERCISES, S.A.F.E. will help a lot of people that have scoliosis and other curvatures, kyphosis and lordosis and help a lot of other youngsters to prevent them from developing scoliosis.

It is my hope that the government or other organization that have the funds and the human resources will contact a research to prove how effective my designed exercises are in treating and preventing the abnormal curvatures of the spine, scoliosis, kyphosis and lordosis.

With the technological means we have these days the research can be done over the internet over a period of six months to a year. There are millions of youngsters diagnosed with scoliosis of various degrees every year.

Take 10,000 youngsters that are diagnosed with scoliosis and instead of advising them "to wait and see "in six months or a year , divide them into   5 groups

1) The first group of 2000 youngsters, just advise them to wait and see what happen in a year ,nothing else .

THIS IS THE STANDARD ADVISE THEY GIVE THE YOUNGSTERS NOW!

2) the second group of 2000 youngsters advised them to just change their postural positional lifestyle.. and start to sit properly while at school and home, avoid slouching positions while watching television for the next six months to a year.

3) the third group of 2000 youngsters advise them to avoid their bad positions lifestyle and start doing the S.A.F.E. exercises I designed based on the Adams forward bend test of the spine, the repeated flexion of the spine without gravity., lying face up while they do the exercises.

4) the fourth group of 2000 youngsters advised them to avoid their bad positioning habits, start doing the exercises I designed S.A.F.E. and add swimming and monkey bar stretching exercises

5) the fifth group of 2000 youngsters after they are diagnosed with scoliosis just advise them to do only the S.A.F.E. exercises daily for six months to a year.

At the end of six months OR one year, check

the x-rays of the youngsters and see which group of youngsters have any improvement in their abnormal scoliosis curve and which group stay the same and which group got worse.

THE RESULTS WILL SPEAK FOR THEMSELVES.

My prediction is:

that group one their scoliosis will get worse, ;they did nothing to help their scoliosis, and they will be doing exactly what they have bee doing to cause the scoliosis in the first place. So unless something dramatic changed in their daily lifestyle habits they will have a worse condition in their spinal curvature.

Group 2 their scoliosis might be the same or have some improvement. At least they changed their bad postural habits, provided they did.

Group 3 their scoliosis should show a lot of improvement and even reverse somewhat. They changed their bad postural habits plus they were doing the S.A.F.E. EXERCISES which are very good in strengthening their spinal muscles and increase their spinal flexibility.

Group 4 of youngsters their scoliosis should improve a lot and even reverse to almost normal depending on how bad it was when they started and how often they do the exercises.

This is the ideal situation for the prevention and treatment of scoliosis.

Group 5 of youngsters should have some improvement but not as much as much as group 4 which , they stopped the bad habits and they were doing swimming and monkey bar exercises.

The S.A.F.E exercises are very good for prevention and treatment of scoliosis but with the complementary exercises of the monkey bar exercises and swimming you get better results in a shorter period of time.

Considering the huge amounts of money that every year the governments and other organizations spend, trying to find a cure for scoliosis ,this research will be easy and cheap to carry out as it can be done over the internet no matter where the youngsters are.

Consider also the huge amounts of money that will be saved by the governments and the patients, if the cure for scoliosis, or just to stop the progression of the spinal abnormal curve is just to do home the S.A.F.E. exercises ,THE MONKEY BAR AND SWIMMING and nothing else,

NO UNCOMFORTABLE BRACES OR RISKY SURGERY OR OTHER EXPENSIVE AND TIME CONSUMING THERAPIES.

Wouldn't that be wonderful for the youngsters and all the people that suffer from scoliosis?

THE FUTURE WILL PROVE IF THE "ADAMS FORWARD BEND" TEST AND THE S.A.F.E. EXERCISES I DESIGNED BASED ON THAT OBSERVATION IS THE MAGIC SOLUTION WE HAVE BEEN LOOKING FOR SO LONG TO HELP THE PEOPLE WITH SCOLIOSIS ,

GIVE THEM A TRY

AND DON'T RUSH TO dismiss them.

MILLIONS OF ATHLETES AND OTHER PEOPLE EXERCISING DAILY DOING SOME OF MY EXERCISES OR SIMILAR EXERCISES IN THEIR DAILY ROUTINE ALONG WITH SWIMMING THE MONKEY BAR OR BODY BUILDING EXERCISES, HAVE STRONG, HEALTHY AND FLEXIBLE SPINES WITHOUT ANY ABNORMAL SPINAL CURVES!

I SIMPLY LIKE TO DRAW THE ATTENTION TO ANYONE THAT HAS SCOLIOSIS OR DIAGNOSES AND TREATS PEOPLE WITH SCOLIOSIS THAT EXERCISES IS A GOOD OPTION TO PREVENT AND TREAT SCOLIOSIS.

IT IS 100% BETTER OPTION THAN THE ONE THAT THEY GIVE TO PEOPLE NOW WHEN THEY FIRST ARE DIAGNOSED

WITH SCOLIOSIS, THE SO CALLED " WAIT AND SEE WHAT HAPPENS IN SIX MONTHS OR A YEAR"

I KNOW THAT MY DESIGNED EXERCISES S.A.F.E. WILL MAKE ANY SPINE STRONGER, FLEXIBLE AND STOP THE PROGRESSION OF SCOLIOSIS PROVIDED THAT PEOPLE WILL DO THEM EVERY DAY............

BUT WHAT IF THE S.A.F.E. EXERCISES ALSO REVERSE COMPLETELY SOME FORMS OF SCOLIOSIS SUCH AS THE FUNCTIONAL SCOLIOSIS AND HELP SOMEWHAT ALL TYPES OF SCOLIOSIS, KYPHOSIS AND LORDOSIS AND MAKE THE LIVES OF PEOPLE BETTER?

DON'T YOU THINK THAT IT IS WORTH INVESTIGATING THAT POSSIBILITY WITH RESEARCH?

The solution to this preventable condition known as SCOLIOSIS, is prevention with good postural habits at home at school, at work and daily exercising to have a strong, flexible and healthy spine.

The SPARTANS of ancient Greece proved that with their well trained soldiers. the BODY BUILDERS and the trained athletes that exercise everyday PROVE IT IN OUR TIMES.

I think it is about time to examine and learn from history what worked well to prevent scoliosis in the past and learn from the present times from the trained athletes that exercise daily and the avoid and prevent the abnormal spinal curves , scoliosis, kyphosis and lordosis.

CHAPTER THIRTEEN

PREVENTION OF SCOLIOSIS

There is a saying that "an once of prevention is worth a ton of therapy."

The best way to prevent scoliosis is exercise, the right exercises and avoid what causes scoliosis which can start as early as soon as a child is born.

As soon as a child is born the doctors and nurses that look after the mother and the child they should give the right instructions to the mother and those that are going to care for the baby how to look after the baby. instructions how to hold the baby to avoid the beginning of scoliosis to the mother and baby. NOT TO HOLD THE BABY ON ONE SIDE OF HER BODY, CAUSING SCOLIOSIS TO HER AND HER BABY.

NEVER TO PUT THE BABY FACE DOWN TO SLEEP,

HAVE THE BABY SLEEP ON HIS BACK OR HIS SIDE

BUT NEVER ALWAYS ONE SIDE, TO AVOID THE MALFORMATION OF THE BABY'S FACE OR SKULL.

BECAUSE THE BONES OF HIS SKULL ARE STILL SOFT

NEVER TO LET OTHER KIDS TO HOLD THE BABY,

THEY MIGHT DROP THE BABY CAUSING INJURIES ETC AND MIGHT CAUSE STRAINS TO THE OTHER KIDS SPINE STARTING A SCOLIOSIS TO THE KIDS.

The parents should take good care of their babies and if they notice an abnormality to their face, spine, hips or legs should take them to their doctor for examination and advice.

The parents should teach their kids by example how to sit properly at the dinner table, while they study, or watching television, or playing video games. They should encourage the kids from young age to exercise more by taking them walking in the park, bicycling, swimming and other activities.

I WAS SURPRISED BUT VERY PLEASED TO SEE RECENTLY ON TELEVISION A PEDIATRICIAN GIVING A YOUNG MOTHER A PRESCRIPTION FOR HER CHILD ' TO DO MORE EXERCISES". I HOPE THIS IS THE NEW TREND AND ALL PEDIATRICIANS WILL GIVE SUCH PRESCRIPTIONS TO ALL THE MOTHERS FOR THEIR KIDS.

Kids should learn from an early age that exercises are good and necessary for good health!

If their kids are diagnosed with scoliosis and they were told to wait and see how it will develop they should encourage them to do the exercises above, enroll them in swimming classes 1-2 times a week and use of a monkey bar to stretch their spine.

If they wait and see the possibility of the abnormal spine will get worse and might need braces and even surgery?

The teachers by example should encourage the kids to sit properly while they sit in the classroom.

The schools should have playgrounds with monkey bars and encourage the kids to use them.

The schools should have at least one session of spinal exercises like the ones I described above every day for 15-20 minutes.

I put a lot of emphasis on the school system, because their students spend a lot of time in schools sitting all day in classes and if they sit in slouching positions and do no exercises there is a possibility that they will get an abnormal postural scoliosis.

Schools should have a scoliosis screening of their students at the beginning and end of each year.

The screening can be done by the school nurse or the gym teacher. A simple plumb line and the Adams's bending forward test will be enough to do the screening and if a scoliosis is detected, or suspected, to refer the student to their doctor. Any students that are diagnosed with scoliosis should do the S.A.F.E. exercises I designed above or similar exercises with swimming and the monkey bar stretching exercises.

It is my understanding, from reading the articles in the dangerous curve,:" A Dangerous Curve: The Role of History in America's ,"other industrialized nations (e.g., Canada, Great Britain, and Australia) that have overturned the

long tradition of mandatory spinal screening of its school-aged citizens.4 ''
that Australia, Canada , England and many states in the United States and other nations discontinued the scoliosis screening in schools because they had complaints about the screening process and that they did not have any benefit in continuing the scoliosis screening.

In the dangerous curve ,there was a picture of a woman with a pen and a clipboard sitting in front of an almost nude girl doing the Adams test and I was wondering what the hell that woman was doing and if she had any training to do the Adams test? That woman was violating the privacy of that girl by having her exposed her underdeveloped chest and if that's how they were conducting the Adams test to all the young girls, I think there were many complaints from the young girls and their parents and rightly so.

The Adams test is done standing behind the child doing the test to observe the spine and not sitting in frond of the child, and in the case of the girls, have them wear a gown or just their shirt backwards to expose only their spine, that's what you are testing.

As for the tests effectiveness and not getting the desirable results to prevent or treat scoliosis I have to agree that the test is only for identify the scoliosis and not to prevent or treat scoliosis.

After you identify the abnormal curve, you have to identify the cause of the abnormal curve and have a program in place to remove the cause and with spinal exercises, swimming and the monkey bar to stop the progression of Scoliosis curve.

If you do nothing and you just wait and see the scoliosis will get worse, no matter if you have the screening for scoliosis in school by doing the Adams test.

You have to use the Adams test to identify the abnormal spinal curve, and implement the program for preventing and correcting the scoliosis with exercises and redo the test periodically to see if the treatments are effective.

For the prevention of scoliosis,

I recommend that all youngsters age 7-18, and EVEN YOUNGER, exercise daily, and this is good for anyone else who wants to have a strong, healthy and flexible spine without any abnormal spinal curves.

The exercises I recommend are: from the
S.A.F.E. EXERCISES

1) SPINAL STRETCH WHILE LYING DOWN FACE UP.

EXTEND YOUR HANDS ABOVE YOUR HEAD TRYING
TO REACH AS FAR AS YOU CAN
AND SIMULTANEOUSLY
WITH YOUR FEET TOGETHER TOUCHING THE
MATTRESS STRETCH THEM DOWN AS FAR AS
YOU CAN

THIS IS A SPINAL STRETCH EXERCISE
FEEL THE SPINAL STRETCH

3) SPINAL STRETCH RAISING YOUR HEAD TOWARDS YOUR CHEST

WHILE SUPPORTING YOUR HEAD WITH YOUR HANDS

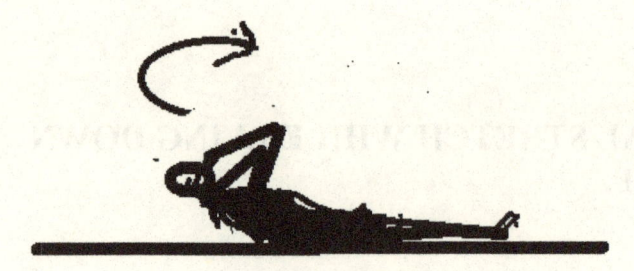

RAISE YOUR HEAD TO YOUR CHEST AS MUCH AS YOU CAN WITHOUT STRAINING YOURSELF,
AND THEN LET YOUR HEAD AND HANDS GENTLY DOWN TO THE MATTRESS.

9) KNEES TO CHEST EXERCISE

**REPEAT THIS EXERCISE
5-10 TIMES**

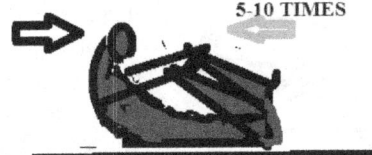

WITH YOUR KNEES BENT DRAW BOTH KNEES TO YOUR CHEST,
GRAB YOUR KNEES WITH BOTH HANDS DRAWING THE KNEES AS NEAR
TO THE CHEST AS POSSIBLE.
AND THEN RAISE YOUR HEAD TOWARDS YOUR KNEES

WITHOUT STRAINING YOURSELF

HOLD IT FOR THE COUNT OF TWO

THEN LOWER YOUR HEAD GENTLY TO THE MATTRESS
AND YOUR FEET TO THE MATTRESS

10)KNEES TO CHEST ROCKING EXERCISE

Knees to chest rocking exercises : this is the most important exercise to increase the flexibility of your spine.

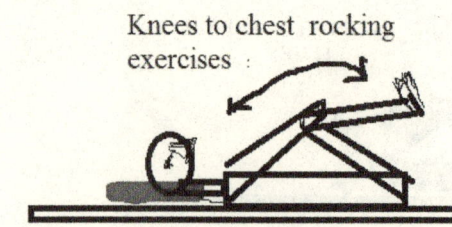

grab your right knee with your right hand and your left knee with your left hand and bring your knees to your chest and with a rocking motion rock your pelvis back and forth

The modified Adam's forward bend exercise

START WITH THE STANDING POSITION BUT
YOUR FEET ARE PLACED 12-18 INCHES APART
BEND FORWARDS AND TOUCH YOUR LEFT
FOOT WITH YOUR RIGHT HAND FINGERS
WHILE YOUR LEFT HAND RESTS ON THE BACK
OF YOUR LOW BACK

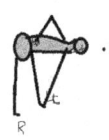

The monkey bar exercise

EXERCISING
ON THE
MONKEY BAR

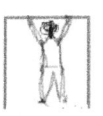

And swimming.
If you do not have access to swimming you can mimic the moves of swimming with standing up, your feet about 18 inches apart and move your right hand all the way up towards to the ceiling and the left hand move backwards as far as you can reach and keep changing their position, one hand up and the other back…… for 3 to 5 minutes.

If you have time and do all the S.A.FE. Exercises every morning when you wake up that's even better.

Always remember that prevention is better than trying to cure it!

GET INTO THE HABIT TO DO THE EXERCISES WHEN YOU WAKE UP IN THE MORNING IN YOUR BED BEFORE YOU GET UP.

CHAPTER FOURTEEN

THINGS TO DO THAT ARE GOOD FOR THE SPINE

1) ALWAYS SIT STRAIGHT WHEN YOU READ, WORK ON THE COMPUTER, IN CLASS AT SCHOOL AND ESPECIALLY WHEN YOU WATCH TV OR MOVIES............

NEVER SLOUCH ON THE SOFA

2) DO GET UP AND MOVE AROUND OFTEN, STANDING OR SITTING TOO LONG STRESSES THE SPINE

3) PLAY SPORTS, SWIMMING, SOCCER, And VOLLEY BALL BUT DO NOT OVERDO IT…..!

4) DANCING IS OK BUT NO DIPS OR WILD MOVES OR AWKWARD HUGGING.

DANCING IS GOOD FOR YOUR MIND AND BODY.

IT IS A GOOD RELAXING EXERCISE

BUT DO NOT OVER DO IT!

5) TRY TO SLEEP ON YOUR BACK IF NOT TRY TO SWITCH SIDES DURING THE NIGHT FROM LEFT TO RIGHT AND VICE VERSA

CHAPTER FIFTEEN

THINGS TO AVOID THAT ARE BAD FOR YOUR SPINE

1) DO NOT SLEEP ON YOUR STOMACH, Although the face down position WOULD BE very good for relaxing and even sleep if the mattress makers made a perfect hole in their mattresses for the face while lying face down, like the hole the massage tables have.
But with the regular mattresses we have now it is not a good idea to sleep face down as it put a lot of twisting pressure on the upper back and especially on the neck and can cause scoliosis on the thoracic cervical(neck) area, other health problems, like headaches, neck pain, shoulder and arm pain.

2) DO NOT RUN FOR LONG DISTANCE UNLESS YOU ARE TRAINED AND HAVE THE NECESSARY GEAR, LIKE PROPER RUNNING SHOES.

3) DO NOT PLAY ON THE TRAMPOLINE, YOU CAN HURT YOURSELF ., UNLESS YOU HAVE PROPER TRAINING

4) NO HEAVY LIFTING AND ALWAYS BEND YOUR KNEES WHEN YOU PICK UP SOMETHING EVEN A PEN…

5) DO NOT CARRY HEAVY OBJECTS OR OVERLOADED BACKPACKS……..AND NEVER CARRY YOUR BACK ON ONE SIDE OF YOUR BODY EVEN IF IT IS NOT HEAVY, THIS FORCES YOUR SPINE INTO A SCOLIOTIC CURVE …

6) AVOID BAD SITTING POSITIONS WHEN YOU READ, WORK ON THE COMPUTER, AT SCHOOL AND ESPECIALLY WHEN YOU WATCH TV OR MOVIES………

BAD SITTING CAUSES A LOT OF HEALTH PROBLEMS INCLUDING SCOLIOSIS AND OTHER POSTURAL PROBLEMS

7) IF YOU HAVE YOUNGER SIBLINGS OR NIECES AND NEPHEWS DO NO LIFT OR HOLD THEM ON ONE SIDE OF YOUR BODY, AS THIS MIGHT BE THE CAUSE OF

SCOLIOSIS…………..

IF YOU BABY-SIT DO NOT LIFT KIDS OR BABIES AND NEVER EVER HOLD BABIES ON ONE SIDE OF YOUR BODY.

8) NO HORSING AROUND OR PLAYING PRACTICAL JOKES ON OTHERS AND IN RETURN THEY PLAY PRACTICAL JOKES ON YOU, THIS CAN CAUSE INJURIES TO YOUR SPINE AND CAUSE A SCOLIOTIC CURVE.

MANY PEOPLE WERE INJURED AND HAD CATASTROPHIC INJURIES FROM HORSING AROUND AND PRACTICAL JOKES.

9) AVOID CONTACT SPORTS LIKE FOOTBALL, WRESTLING AND HOCKEY.

The practice of targeting the good players of the other team, to injure them and get them off the game so that the other team win, SHOULD BE OUTLAWED AND CRIMINALIZED. I was appalled, shocked and dismayed while watching hockey on television to see a player attack the best player of the opposite team from behind and driving the head of that payer on the ice causing him serious injuries. That's AN INTENTIONAL CRIMINAL assault causing serious injuries and should be recognized as such ,outlawed , frowned upon such acts and proper punishment ,like jail time and ban from playing that sport.

The motto should be ,' may the best player win fair and square.", and not "lets injure him so that we win." Kids that are watching will try to do it too and that's very dangerous.!

10)AVOID EXCESSIVE HUGGING ESPECIALLY WHEN YOUR BODY IS IN AN AWKWARD POSITION .IF YOU HAVE TO HUG, YOUR BODY SHOULD BE STRAIGHT AND FACING THE ONE YOU HUG. AVOID SIDE HUGS OR VIOLENT HUGS LIKE THE "BEAR HUG"
IF YOU DO NOT FEEL LIKE HUGGING SOMEBODY , YOU DO NOT HAVE TO HUG ANYONE, JUST PUT YOUR ARM IN FRONT OF YOU AND TELL THE INDENTED HUGGER THAT YOU ARE NOT A HUGGER. IT AS SIMPLE AS THAT!

CHAPTER SIXTEEN

KEEP A DAILY DIARY.

WHEN YOU START DOING THE S.A.F.E.
SPINAL EXERCISES
KEEP A DAILY DIARY.

TAKE A PICTURE OF YOUR SPINE JUST
BEFORE STARTING THE EXERCISES AND
RETAKE PICTURES OF YOUR SPINE
EVERY WEEK TO SEE THE PROGRESS YOU
ARE MAKING.
YOU SHOULD SEE SOME IMPROVEMENTS
IN YOUR SPINE IN 4-6 WEEKS AND AS
TIME GOES BYE, YOU WILL HAVE A
STRONGER, HEALTHIER, MORE FLEXIBLE
SPINE AND THE ABNORMAL CURVE
REDUCED.

EVERY DAY WRITE DOWN EXACTLY HOW
YOU DO THE EXERCISES, HOW MANY
TIMES YOU DO EACH EXERCISE   AND
HOW YOU FEEL AFTER THE EXERCISES.
REMEMBER NEVER TO STRAIN YOURSELF
AND AS YOU GET STRONGER   INCREASE
THE REPETITIONS OF EACH EXERCISE.

THE DAILY DIARY WILL MOTIVATE AND ECOURAGE YOU WHEN YOU START SEEING IMPROVEMENTS IN YOUR SCOLIOSIS.

AS TIME GOES BYE AND YOU FEEL STRONGER, YOU INCREASE THE NUMBER OF EXERCISES YOU DO.
MORE REPETITIONS MEAN STRONGER MUSCLES AND MORE FLEXIBLE SPINE.

THE MOST IMPORTANT THING IS THAT YOU DO THESE EXERCISES DAILY AND AVOID ANYTHING THAT AGREVATES YOUR SCOLIOSIS WHICH I DESCRIBE ABOVE ON   CHAPTER FIFTEEN   " THINGS TO AVOID"

CHAPTER SEVENTEEN.

IF YOU OR YOUR CHILD IS DIAGNOSED WITH SCOLIOSIS.

If you or your child is diagnosed with scoliosis, you should know that you are not the only one suffering from this condition. Unfortunately, there are millions of people suffering from this condition.

Many doctors called it "IDIOPATHIC SCOLIOSIS" MEANING THAT THEY DO NOT KNOW WHAT IS CAUSING YOUR SCOLIOSIS. However if they do not know the cause of your scoliosis it does not mean that there is no cause, it is simply that they did not figure out the cause yet, but there is always A CAUSE, for scoliosis,

From an old injury that was not reported or diagnosed and treated properly to a simple carrying your child or other heavy objects such as heavy handbags on one side of your body, or just slouching on your favorite sofa watching television. There are many causes for scoliosis, not just one cause.

No matter what was the cause of your scoliosis, which you and your doctors do not know, you have to know that there is a way to help yourself or your child to get better with the spinal active flexion exercises(S.A.F.E.)Which I describe above in this book.

Unfortunately there is no magic pill to take and make the scoliosis disappear but with the spinal exercises you and your child will have a good chance to stop the progression of the abnormal

curve and even reverse it back to a healthy spine. Do not expect miracles to happen overnight , but if you have the will, desire and determination to do the exercises daily in the privacy of your home in your own bed or just a mat on the floor of your house, you will have a good chance get a strong and healthy spine.
I designed these exercises based on the observation that millions of athletes that exercise daily with similar exercises have a strong, healthy spine without scoliosis or any other abnormal curves and they have a good posture that is the envy of many people.
I also based my exercises on the Adam's forward bend test in which a scoliotic spine straightens when you bend your spine.

So I combined the observation made by Williams Adams for his famous "the Adams test" and my observation how athletes get strong healthy spines and you have the Spinal active flexion exercises which will give you and anybody else with scoliosis no matter what caused that scoliosis the opportunity to have a strong and healthy spine.

If you or your child want to get better, You have to do the exercises; NOBODY ELSE CAN DO IT FOR YOU.
IT IS YOUR CHOICE, you do the exercises and you get better or you do nothing and you get

worse.
 So far "the wait and see approach" used by many health professionals did not work well for the people suffering from scoliosis and many end up with surgery and rods in their spine.

CHAPTER EIGHTEEN

IF YOU ARE A HEALTH PROFESSIONAL TREATING PEOPLE WITH SCOLIOSIS.

I am sure you are doing your best to help your patients and I commend you for that . Many times you are frustrated or disappointed for not getting as good results with your procedures as you wish to get.
As you know, SCOLIOSIS is called IDIOPATHIC, meaning that there is no known cause for the abnormal spinal curve and by not knowing the cause, the treatments are not effective.
However scoliosis has not only one cause but many causes and you have to do some detective work to find the possible cause of each individuals scoliosis, name it accordingly and when you know what the cause is by simply removing the cause the patient will get better.
Take for example the idiopathic infantile scoliosis which is most likely caused by the bad position the hold or have the child sleep and many times affects the face and the malformation of the skull , it should be called POSITIONAL INFANTILE SCOLIOSIS , because it is caused by the bad position they hold or position the child. It is like we call the cervical strain from a car accident, WHIPLASH, and not a simple neck strain or injury so that everyone who treats that patient knows the cause

and take the necessary precautions.
I think the health professionals should reclassify the idiopathic scoliosis according to its cause.
If there is a true short leg, which is the foundation of the human body, no treatment can help the scoliosis of that patient unless you correct the short leg with a shoe or heel lift. So it is appropriate to call that type of scoliosis A TRUE SHORT LEG SCOLIOSIS and not IDIOPATHIC SCOLIOSIS because idiopathic scoliosis does not tell us where the problem is but the true short leg scoliosis tell us exactly what is causing the scoliosis and how to correct it.
In my book I describe some of the possible causes of scoliosis and suggestions how to treat each type of scoliosis by removing the underlying cause first and then do the specific spinal exercises to strengthen the spinal muscles to correct the curves.

I designed my SPINAL ACTIVE FLEXION EXERCISES S.A.F.E. based on the Adam's forward bend test in which a scoliotic spine straightens when you bend your spine and my observation how millions of athletes exercising daily have healthy spines without any abnormal curves.
So I combined the observation made by Williams Adams for his famous "the Adams test" and my observation how athletes get strong healthy spines and you have the Spinal

active flexion exercises which will give you and anybody else with scoliosis no matter what caused that scoliosis the opportunity to have a strong and healthy spine.

It is my hope that the health professionals will re-examine and re-name and reclassify the so called IDIOPATHIC SCOLIOSIS according to the possible cause of each individuals scoliosis ,instead of the now known name IDIOPATHIC SCOLIOSIS regardless of what the cause is.

It is also my hope that the professionals that treat people with scoliosis will recognize the value of the spinal exercises in treating the abnormal curves and encourage their patients to start spinal corrective exercises for the prevention and treatment of scoliosis, especially when it is diagnosed in the early stage of scoliosis.

The solution to prevent and treat scoliosis is daily exercises.
In severe scoliosis the surgery and rods is the best choice but by encouraging the people with mild to moderate scoliosis to exercise daily might help them to avoid surgery.

Braces or casting might be necessary when there is a fracture, or severe injury but for early stages of scoliosis the exercise are by far the better choice.

The millions of people that exercise daily prove that. They have strong healthy and flexible spines and no scoliosis.
I hope that you will encourage your patients to try my designed exercises along with whatever you are now doing so that you will get better results for your patients.

CHAPTER NINETEEN

CONCLUSION

Considering the human suffering and the huge

amounts of money spend in this preventable disease, the scoliosis,
I hope that the health professionals that first diagnose this condition will advice their patients what to do to avoid the progression of the curve, avoid expensive treatments and risky surgeries, by giving them a copy of my designed exercises, S.A.F.E.

'what's good for your spine' and

'what to avoid to have a good strong spine."

It is obvious that the status quo ,
'" of wait and see approach", is not working and many youngsters end up using spinal braces and risky surgeries .

It is also my hope that governments and schools will have an active role in screening for scoliosis and encourage youngsters to exercise more during school hours, like many companies do with their workers providing exercise time during working hours to prevent scoliosis , and provide ergonomic desks and chairs
There is no magic pill and never will be any magic pill to correct the spinal curves but with exercises you can keep your spine in good shape and without abnormal curves.

To have a strong, flexible and healthy spine you have to exercise daily to have strong spinal muscles.

Athletes that exercise daily, like body builders, swimmers runners and others, have strong healthy spines and rarely if ever get any abnormal spinal curves like scoliosis.

THE SPINAL ACTIVE FLEXION EXERCISES (S.A.F.E.) I DESIGNED WILL HELP PEOPLE WITH SCOLIOSIS AND OTHER SPINAL CURVATURES TO GET A FLEXIBLE, STRONGER HEALTHIER SPINE

AND EVEN IF A FRACTION OF THE MILLIONS OF YOUNGSTERS WITH SCOLIOSIS ARE HELPED WITH THE OBSERVATION OF WILLIAMS ADAMS AND MY DESIGNED EXERCISES, THIS BOOK WILL ACCOMPLISH ITS PURPOSE:

TO HELP AS MANY PEOPLE WITH SCOLIOSIS AS POSSIBLE.

If you or any of your family and kids is diagnosed with scoliosis and" told to wait and see," instead of waiting in anguish what will happen down the road in six months or a year, give my S.A.F.E. exercises a try with the blessing of your health provider. You have nothing to loose and at least your are doing something about it and don't be surprised if the scoliosis reverse itself or at least does not progress.

Good luck to every one and may god bless the exercises you will be doing and eliminate your spinal problems!

CHAPTER TWENTY

EPILOGUE

I never thought that I will be writing this book. However the prospect that my designed exercises will help even a fraction of the millions of people that are suffering from SCOLIOSIS, and with the help of KDP I did it.

It is my desire and wish that all those who will DO my designed exercises daily will benefit a lot and prove that I did the right thing to design and publish my SPINAL ACTIVE FLEXION

EXERCISES (S.A.F.E.)

It is my hope that with exercises and preventative education on how youngsters can take good care of their spines and proper treatments, will eliminate this preventable disease named SCOLIOSIS.(crooked spine)

My greatest satisfaction will be when these exercises help people with scoliosis, to have a strong, healthy flexible spine with less spinal curvatures and have a healthier life.

THE AUTHOR

S.ELIA

Disclaimer:
This book is for information ONLY and is not intended to serve as medical advice. Anyone seeking specific advice or assistance should consult his or her doctor . if they do not like the advice of their doctor they should seek a second opinion from another doctor.

REFERENCES:

1) A Dangerous Curve: The Role of History in America's Scoliosis Screening Programs

2) ADAMS TEST

BACK BOOK COVER

SCOLIOSIS:

A FRESH LOOK AT WHAT CAUSES THE IDIOPATHIC FUNCTIONAL SCOLIOSIS AND HOME EXERCISES TO STOP THE PROGRESSION OF THE CURVE AND EVEN REVERSE IT BACK TO NORMAL

HOPE TO EVERY MOTHERS ANGUISH FOR HER CHILDS CROOKED SPINE

TRYING TO TAME THE ABNORMAL DANGEROUS CURVES WITH HOME EXERCISES FOR ALL THOSE WHO ARE DIAGNOSED WITH SCOLIOSIS, TO STOP THE PROGRESSION OF THE ABNORMAL SPINAL CURVE AND GET A HEALTHY, FLEXIBLE STRONG SPINE

Scoliosis is the million dollar question? How to prevent it and how to stop the progression of the abnormal spinal curve with home exercises! And the answer is THE SPINAL ACTIVE FLEXION. EXERCISES!!(S.A.F.E.) DONE IN

THE PRIVACY OF YOUR HOME IN YOUR OWN BED!

Made in the USA
Las Vegas, NV
13 March 2024